D1760855

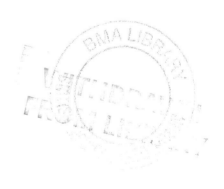

Managing Complications in Glaucoma Surgery

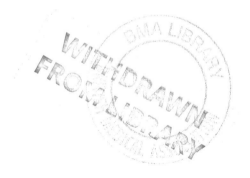

Francis Carbonaro • K. Sheng Lim
Editors

Managing Complications in Glaucoma Surgery

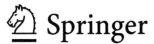 Springer

Editors
Francis Carbonaro, MD, PhD, FRCOphth.
Mater Dei Hospital
Msida
Malta

K. Sheng Lim, MBChB, FRCOphth, MD
St Thomas' Hospital
London
UK

ISBN 978-3-319-49414-2   ISBN 978-3-319-49416-6   (eBook)
DOI 10.1007/978-3-319-49416-6

Library of Congress Control Number: 2017933708

Printed on acid-free paper

This Springer imprint is published by Springer Nature
The registered company is Springer International Publishing AG
The registered company address is: Gewerbestrasse 11, 6330 Cham, Switzerland

Contents

Glaucoma Laser

Jason Cheng, Mariana Cabrera, Jacky W.Y. Lee, and Yvonne M. Buys

1.1 Lasers That Increase Aqueous Outflow: Argon Laser Trabeculoplasty

1.1.1 Introduction

Argon laser trabeculoplasty (ALT) was first introduced in 1979 by Wise and Witter (Coakes 1992). Despite its clinical efficacy in intraocular pressure (IOP) lowering, its use is limited by scarring of the trabecular meshwork, which may potentially restrict retreatment.

1.1.2 Procedure

ALT is usually performed with topical anesthesia under direct visualization using a gonioscopic lens. Initially, only 180° of the meshwork is treated. Around 40–50 laser spots are aimed at the anterior half of the trabecular meshwork to reduce the chance of peripheral anterior synechiae (PAS) formation. The laser spot size is 50 μm and the initial laser energy of 800 mW is titrated until minimal bubble formation in the pigmented trabecular meshwork is seen. After 4–6 weeks, IOP is reassessed and the remaining half of the trabecular meshwork may be treated if needed. Topical steroids are usually given for the first week after ALT (Weinreb and Wilensky 1984).

J. Cheng (✉)
Khoo Teck Puat Hospital, Yishun, Singapore
e-mail: jdcheng@gmail.com

M. Cabrera • Y.M. Buys
Department of Ophthalmology and Vision Sciences, University of Toronto, Toronto, Canada

J.W.Y. Lee
Dennis Lam & Partners Eye Center, Hong Kong, China

F. Carbonaro, K. Sheng Lim (eds.), *Managing Complications in Glaucoma Surgery*,
DOI 10.1007/978-3-319-49416-6_1, © Springer International Publishing AG 2017

1.1.3   Efficacy and Outcomes

In one of the largest randomized controlled trials involving 3608 subjects, comparing ALT versus Timolol 0.5 % as primary treatment for open-angle glaucoma (OAG), ALT lowered the IOP by 9 mmHg compared to a 7 mmHg drop in those using medication alone. At 2 years, 44 % of ALT-treated eyes did not require additional interventions compared to 30 % in the medication group. By 7 years, the ALT group continued to have lower IOPs and less visual field progression compared to the medication group. The authors concluded that ALT had a similar efficacy to Timolol 0.5 % (Glaucoma laser trial 1991). In the literature, the range of IOP reduction is from 13 % to 32 % in OAG eyes (Stein and Challa 2007). In comparison with selective laser trabeculoplasty (SLT), a meta-analysis has concluded that the IOP-lowering effects between the two lasers were similar or at least one was not inferior to the other (Wong et al. 2015).

1.1.4   Complications

1.1.4.1   Intraoperative Complications

Hyphema can occur from inadvertent laser shots to the iris root or as a result of blood reflux from the Schlemm's canal. Pain may be experienced during the laser treatment despite the application of topical anesthetic agents, and vasovagal syncope has been a reported complication of ALT (Weinreb and Wilensky 1984).

1.1.4.2   Early Postoperative Complications

Immediately following ALT treatment, the protein and inflammatory mediator contents in the anterior chamber are increased. As a result of trabecular meshwork blockage by extracellular debris and swelling, the IOP may rise by 5 mmHg in 34 % of patients and up to 10 mmHg in 12 % of patients following treatment (Coakes 1992). The IOP spike usually occurs anywhere from 2 to 4 hours after ALT and is associated with the use of higher laser energies, 360° as opposed to 180° treatments, and more posterior laser applications (Coakes 1992). IOP spikes may be prevented with a topical alpha-adrenergic agent, whereas the control of the inflammation with topical steroids does not seem to alter the course of IOP elevations (Coakes 1992).

A degree of anterior uveitis is present in all patients after ALT, although it is often self-limiting and transient in nature. The prescription of a topical steroid is a common practice after ALT (Coakes 1992).

1.1.4.3   Late Postoperative Complications

Anterior chamber inflammation and too posteriorly placed laser shots may lead to PAS formation, which can occur at an incidence of 12 %–47 % after ALT (Coakes 1992; Weinreb and Wilensky 1984; Wong et al. 2015). In histological analysis of eyes treated with ALT, it was found that the trabecular beams were severely distorted together with the loss of the trabecular endothelial cells and the formation of a cellular sheet that extends from the Schwalbe's line to the anterior aspect of the trabecular meshwork (Coakes 1992).

Other less common late postoperative complications reported in the literature include corneal endothelial damage, unexplained visual field loss in two elderly patients, and even a rare case of presumed sympathetic ophthalmia in an aphakic eye with uveitis at 1 year after ALT (Juhas 1993; Coakes 1992; Weinreb and Wilensky 1984).

1.2   Lasers That Increase Aqueous Outflow: Selective Laser Trabeculoplasty

1.2.1   Introduction

Selective laser trabeculoplasty (SLT) was first described by Latina and Park in 1995. It is performed using a frequency-doubled (Q-switched) Nd:YAG laser (Wong et al. 2015). It selectively targets melanoctyes in the trabecular meshwork and only delivers 1 % of the energy used in the former ALT technology. As SLT does not induce any trabecular meshwork scarring, repeated treatments are possible. In 2001, the United States Food and Drug Administration approved the use of SLT for the treatment of OAG.

1.2.2   Procedure

As with ALT, SLT is performed under topical anesthesia using a gonioscopic lens. An initial energy of 0.8 mJ is used with titration in energy level until bubble formation is just visible in the trabecular meshwork. The laser spot size is 400 μm and the duration is 3 ns. Nonoverlapping laser shots are applied to 180°–360° of the trabecular meshwork. A higher total laser energy has been associated with a greater chance of IOP reduction (Lee et al. 2015). Postoperative eye drops may vary from a weak topical steroid, topical nonsteroidal anti-inflammatory, to no postoperative eye drops.

1.2.3   Efficacy and Outcomes

In a recent meta-analysis of randomized controlled trials on the use of SLT in the treatment of OAG, it was reported that the range of IOP reduction varies from 6.9 to 35.9 % at ≥12 months post-SLT among patients newly diagnosed with glaucoma to those who were already on maximally tolerated topical antiglaucoma medications. Wong et al. concluded that SLT is noninferior to ALT and topical antiglaucoma medication in terms of IOP reduction and achieving treatment success. The amount of medication reduction is also similar between SLT and ALT (Wong et al. 2015). Koucheki et al. reported a similar rate of IOP reduction among primary open-angle glaucoma (POAG), pseudoexfoliation, and pigmentary glaucoma patients; however, those with diabetes had a lower amount of IOP reduction following SLT. Pigmentary glaucoma has been reported to be associated with more complications including significant pressure spikes following SLT; occasionally requiring surgical intervention (Koucheki and Hashemi 2012).

1.2.4 Complications

1.2.4.1 Intraoperative Complications
Throughout the literature, SLT seems to be a relatively safe procedure without many severe intraoperative complications (Wong et al. 2015). Some potential complications during the procedure may include corneal abrasion, subconjunctival hemorrhage, hyphema, and ocular pain. Some patients may experience an ipsilateral headache or photophobia after the laser (Klamann et al. 2014; Wong et al. 2015).

1.2.4.2 Early Postoperative Complications
The majority of side effects of SLT are mild and transient including: anterior uveitis, IOP spikes, conjunctivitis, corneal edema (Fig. 1.1), visual blurring, and only one case report of choroidal effusion and three case reports of cystoid macular edema (Klamann et al. 2014; Wong et al. 2015).

Given the lower energy used in SLT as compared to ALT, the majority of anterior uveitis after SLT settles within 3 to 5 days (Lee et al. 2014a). Koucheki et al. reported an inflammatory rate of 42.6 % in OAG eyes (Koucheki and Hashemi 2012). Jinapriya et al. compared the use of artificial tears, prednisolone acetate 1 %, or ketorolac tromethamine 0.5 % eye drops four times per day for 5 days following SLT and found that the use of an anti-inflammatory medication for a short period of time after SLT did not affect the IOP-lowering efficacy of the laser (Jinapriya et al. 2014).

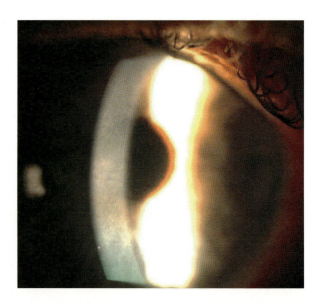

Fig. 1.1 Corneal edema after SLT (Taken from a case report by Moubayed et al. (2009))

Similar to ALT, IOP spikes can occur within 1 to 2 hours of the procedure with spikes >5 mmHg in about 10 % of patients and spikes >10 mmHg in 3 % following SLT (Barkana and Belkin 2007). Similar to ALT, a topical alpha-adrenergic agent may be used as prophylaxis before or immediately after the procedure. However, it should be noted that increased trabecular meshwork pigment has been associated with significant IOP spikes necessitating urgent filtration surgery, thus, lower energies or perhaps less invasive laser trabeculoplasties like MicroPulse Laser Trabeculoplasty (MLT) may be considered in these cases (Koucheki and Hashemi 2012).

1.2.4.3 Late Postoperative Complications

Given the close proximity of the cornea to the trabecular meshwork, potential damage to the cornea following SLT needs to be considered. Moubayed et al. were the first to report a case of permanent corneal edema progressing into bullous keratopathy following SLT (Moubayed et al. 2009).

Knickelbein et al. reported four cases that developed corneal edema and subsequent corneal thinning and hyperopic shift, with two cases requiring contact lens wear. Although the cause of this rare complication remains unknown, it may be associated with myopia (Knickelbein et al. 2014).

Figure 1.2 from Ong and Ong illustrates a marked increase in dark spots/patches on specular microscopy following SLT reported in two patients with pre-SLT corneal pigment. Thus, the corneal endothelium should be examined for pigment deposition, corneal guttatae, or evidence of compromise prior to SLT (Ong and Ong 2013). Lee et al. (2014a) from Hong Kong investigated 111 eyes of 66 Chinese OAG subjects treated with SLT. They measured the endothelial cell count using a

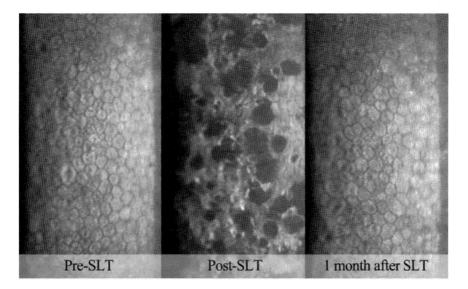

Fig. 1.2 The corneal endothelium of a patient before and after SLT showing a marked increase in dark spots/patches on specular microscopy (Taken from a case report by Ong and Ong (2013))

specular microscopy, central corneal thickness (CCT) videokeratography, and the spherical equivalent using a kerato-refractometer. Readings were taken before and at 1 month after SLT. The intraclass correlation coefficient (0.997) among these investigations was high, signifying excellent reproducibility of these measurements. The mean endothelial cell count was reduced by 4.5 % from baseline (2465.0 ± 334.0 cells/mm^2) at 1 week (2355.0±387.0 cells/mm^2) after SLT (p = 0.0004). At 1 month (2424.0 ± 379.4 cells/mm^2, p = 0.3), the endothelial cell count returned to baseline levels. The authors attributed inflammatory cell attachment and microscopic endothelial cell edema as the causes of the apparent reduction in endothelial cell count as both of these conditions can affect the accuracy of cell counts with specular microscopy. On slit-lamp examination, none of the subjects had any clinically visible corneal edema. In a recent randomized controlled trial that compared SLT versus prostaglandin analogs in the treatment of primary angle closure glaucoma in subjects that had at least 180° of angle opening, the 6-month endothelial cell loss was 4.8 % from baseline (p = 0.001) (Narayanaswamy et al. 2014). This was in contrast to the 4.5 % transient reduction in the study by Lee et al. (2014a). The differences in angle opening among the two study populations could have accounted for the permanent damages documented by Narayanaswamy et al. (2014) since a narrower angle can predispose the corneal endothelium to absorb a greater amount of dissipated laser heat.

In Lee et al.'s study (Lee et al. 2014a), CCT decreased 1.1 % from 549.4 ± 37.6 μm at baseline to 543.9 ± 40.2 μm at 1 week (p = 0.02). By 1 month, CCT was back to baseline level (p = 0.2). Laser heat dissipation could have led to a thermal-induced corneal stromal contraction in the collagen fibers. When the keratocytes get replenished, the CCT returns to its original thickness. There was no evidence of clinically visible scarring on the cornea in the 111 OAG eyes that received SLT treatment. There were also no statistically significant changes in the spherical equivalent following SLT. Thus, in cases with angle closure elements, the potential risks of corneal damage should be discussed with patients prior to treatment.

The rate of peripheral anterior synechia formation following SLT is around 2.86 % or less which is significantly less than that reported after ALT (Wong et al. 2015). Damji et al. published the only randomized controlled trial comparing the safety of ALT versus SLT (Damji et al. 2006). A comparison in the side effects of these two lasers is summarized in Table 1.1. Table 1.2 summarizes complications of SLT reported in a recent meta-analysis (Wong et al. 2015).

Key Points
- Intraocular pressure spikes can occur 1 to 2 hour after the procedure. Topical alpha-adrenergic agent may be used as prophylaxis before or after the procedure.
- Increased trabecular meshwork pigment has been associated with extreme intraocular pressure spikes. Therefore, lower energy with close monitoring is recommended in these patients.

Table 1.1 Comparison of complications between ALT and SLT from a randomized controlled by study by Damji et al. (2006)

Complications	ALT ($n = 87$) (%)	SLT ($n = 89$) (%)
IOP spike > 6 mmHg	3.4	4.5
PAS formation	1.2	1.1
ALT retreatment within 1 year	5.7	3.4
SLT retreatment within 1 year	4.6	6.7
Trabeculectomy within 1 year	8.0	9.0
Glaucoma drainage device within 1 year	0.0	1.1
Cyclophotocoagulation within 1 year	0.0	1.1

PAS peripheral anterior synechiae, *ALT* argon laser trabeculoplasty, *SLT* selective laser trabeculoplasty, *IOP* intraocular pressure

Table 1.2 Frequencies of SLT complications

Complications	Percentage or number of cases
Side effects reported by case series:	
Transient IOP rise	0–62 %
With prophylactic/empirical treatment	0–28.8 %
Anterior chamber inflammation	0–89.3 %
Eye pain/discomfort	0–58 % (up to 65.7 % if redness included)
Peripheral anterior synechiae	0–2.86 %
Headache	4 %
Photophobia	3–96.7 %
Hyphema	0 %
Pigment dispersion	0 %
Conjunctival hyperemia	9–64 %
Corneal haze	0–0.2 %
Corneal abrasion	0.65 %
Corneal endothelial dark/white spots	50 %
Cystoid macular edema	0 %
Side effects from case reports:	
High IOP spikes (IOP 26–65 mmHg)	4 cases
Bilateral anterior uveitis following single eye SLT	1 case
Hyphema	2 cases
Corneal edema/haze/thinning	4 cases
Diffuse lamellar keratitis	1 case
Cystoid macular edema	3 cases
Severe iritis with choroidal effusion	1 case

Taken from a meta-analysis by Wong et al. (2015)

1.3   Lasers That Increase Aqueous Outflow: Micropulse Laser Trabeculoplasty and Titanium-Sapphire Laser Trabeculoplasty

1.3.1   Introduction

MicroPulse Laser Trabeculoplasty (MLT) can be delivered using a diode (810 nm) or a 532 nm/577 nm laser. The MLT technology makes use of a 15 % on and 85 % off duty cycle to minimize the thermal damage to the surrounding tissues. Although ALT causes damage and scarring to the trabecular meshwork and SLT destroys melanocytes through heat, MLT neither destroys nor scars the trabecular meshwork (Fudemberg et al. 2008).

Titanium-sapphire laser trabeculoplasty (TLT) is an emerging subtype of laser trabeculoplasty that uses a 790 nm laser (SOLX, Inc., Waltham, Massachusetts, USA) to emit near-infrared energy in pulses ranging from 5 to 10 ms.

1.3.2   Procedure

Similar to ALT and SLT, MLT is performed under topical anesthesia. However, the gonioscopic lens of MLT has a built-in, visible, inner reference guide that allows the surgeon to deliver exactly 10 confluent laser shots per clock hour for a total of 120 shots over 360°. The spot size is 300 µm, treatment duration 300 ms, and an initial power of 1000 mW. There are no visible endpoints in MLT, hence, the energy is only titrated down if the patient experiences pain during the procedure. No anti-inflammatory medications are required after MLT.

For TLT, the wavelength is 690 nm with energies of 30–80 mJ at pulse duration of 7 ms. The spot size is smaller than SLT or ALT at 200 µm. The laser is aimed at the pigmented trabecular meshwork and 50 nonoverlapping shots may be applied to 180° of the pigmented trabecular meshwork. The endpoint is the formation of bubbles or the visible bursting of pigments from the trabecular meshwork.

1.3.3   Efficacy and Outcomes

Gossage reported the 2-year data after treatment of 532 nm MLT in 18 POAG eyes. Three laser energies of 300 mW, 700 mW, and 1000 mW were used and at 4 months, those receiving 1000 mW had the greatest amount of IOP reduction of 30 %. At 24 months, the amount of IOP reduction in the group receiving 1000 mW treatment was 24 % (Gossage 2015).

There are very few studies reporting the efficacy of TLT. A 15-month pilot study with 37 subjects, reported that TLT-treated eyes had a mean IOP reduction of 32 % as compared to 25 % in the ALT group (Goldenfeld et al. 2009).

1.3.4 Complications

1.3.4.1 Intraoperative Complications

There are no reported intraoperative complications from MLT in the literature. In theory, the risk of intraoperative bleeding and pain should be less than in ALT and SLT due to the shorter duration of laser action from the duty cycle technology.

1.3.4.2 Early Postoperative Complications

Fea et al. (2008) reported on the safety of the 810 nm MLT in 32 eyes of 20 patients with OAG. The inferior 180° of the trabecular meshwork was treated and a Kowa FM 500 flare-meter was used to measure anterior chamber reaction at baseline and at 3 h, 1 day, 1 week, and 12 months after MLT. Only one patient (5 %) was found to have an increase in flare after MLT. The same patient, who had a history of pigmentary glaucoma, developed an IOP spike of 34 mmHg requiring oral acetazolamide treatment for 2 days. Otherwise, MLT was well tolerated apart from burning or heat sensation that was reported in four (20 %) of the patients.

In a prospective series in Hong Kong by Lee et al. using a 577 nm MLT in the treatment of OAG, only 7.5 % of treated OAG eyes had a mild and self-limiting anterior uveitis that resolved without medication. There was no corneal edema detected on slit-lamp examination and no recorded IOP spikes at day 1, 1 week, or 1 month after MLT (data pending publication). As MLT is still a relatively new technology; only gaining popularity in the early 2010s, larger-scale, randomized studies are warranted before its long-term safety in comparison with its predecessors can be determined.

For TLT, the IOP spike rate has been reported to be around 11 %.

1.3.4.3 Late Postoperative Complications

At present, the longest study involving the use of MLT in OAG is 2 years. There are no reported late postoperative complications in the literature (Fudemberg et al. 2008).

In a study of 18 patients with OAG treated with TLT, none of the patients developed PAS nor were there any reported long-term complications over a 2-year period.

1.4 Lasers That Increase Angle Width: Laser Peripheral Iridotomy

1.4.1 Introduction

Angle closure glaucoma is an optic neuropathy secondary to raised intraocular pressure (IOP) due to closure of the drainage angle. A number of different factors contribute to primary angle closure, including pupillary block, thickened iris root, cataract, and plateau iris configuration. Peripheral iridotomy removes the pupillary block mechanism by allowing aqueous to flow from the posterior chamber to the anterior chamber, by-passing the pupil. Laser peripheral iridotomy (LPI) has now essentially replaced the surgical iridectomy.

LPI is indicated for acute primary angle closure, the fellow eye in acute primary angle closure glaucoma if the angle is felt to be occludable, primary angle closure (angle closure with evidence of peripheral anterior synechia or raised IOP, but no glaucomatous optic neuropathy), primary angle closure glaucoma (primary angle closure with glaucomatous optic neuropathy) and primary angle closure suspects (angle closure in at least two quadrants of trabecular meshwork without any of the above findings). There is some evidence that LPI can be helpful in phacomorphic glaucoma and pigment dispersion syndrome.

1.4.2 Procedure

Table 1.3 summarizes the technique of LPI. The iridotomy needs to be of sufficient size to allow aqueous flow and pressure equalization between the anterior and posterior chambers. Mathematical modeling using Navier–Stokes equations suggests that a peripherial iridotomy length of 50 μm would reduce the pressure differential to under 1 mmHg (Silver and Quigley 2004). It has been proposed that a minimum diameter of at least 150 μm is necessary to add in a safety margin to account for posttreatment iris edema, fibrosis, pigment epithelial proliferation, or pupil dilation (Fleck 1990).

Table 1.3 Recommendations on technique of performing laser peripheral iridotomy (LPI) at different stages

Stage of procedure	Recommendations on technique of performing LPI
Pretreatment	Constrict pupil with 1–4 % pilocarpine 3 drops over 10–30 min Topical anesthesia such as tetracaine or alcaine
Treatment	Use iridotomy contact lens such as Abraham (+66D button) or Wise (+103D button) Placement of iridotomy at either side of 12 o'Clock or just above or below 3 or 9 o'clock
Optional pretreatment – argon laser for dark iris	Stage 1: spot size 50um, duration 0.1 s, power 100–200 mW around 15–25 shots Stage 2: spot size 50um, duration 0.1 s, power 500–700 mW around 15–25 shots
Nd:YAG settings	Power: 1–5 mJ Spot size and duration is fixed
Posttreatment	A single dose of topical Brimonidine 0.2 % and steroid may be administered to reduce postlaser pressure spike and inflammation Topical steroids can be prescribed 4 times a day for 1 week IOP should be checked 1 h after LPI Iridotomy should be checked for size and patency Gonioscopy should be repeated to document change in angle post iridotomy

1.4.3   Complications

1.4.3.1   During Laser Iridotomy Procedure

Bubbles may form during the laser and may obstruct the visualization of the iridotomy site. The size and likelihood of bubbles is related to the argon laser power. Therefore, starting with a lower power, then increasing the power in stage 2 is recommended (see Table 1.3) (de Silva et al. 2007). The 12 o'clock position for LPI placement should be avoided as this is where bubbles congregate. If bubbles form they are absorbed rapidly and are of no consequence.

Argon laser corneal epithelium burns manifest as milky white spots, whereas corneal endothelial burns appear as opacities. Nd:YAG laser injury to the cornea appears as star-shaped bursts. These corneal injuries occur due to poor focusing. A mobile eye, shallow anterior chamber, or cloudy cornea can increase the risk of corneal injury. In the event of an injury, the procedure may need to be abandoned or a new LPI location chosen where the anterior chamber is deeper and there is less corneal clouding. Corneal epithelial burns recover after 1–2 days. Direct endothelial cell damage is not reversible but usually remains localized. Routine LPI for primary angle closure suspects does not appear to increase the risk of endothelial cell loss. A Singaporean study comparing the endothelial cell count after LPI to the fellow untreated eye found that both groups had a reduced endothelial cell count (3.6 % and 3.2 %, respectively) at 3 years, but the difference between both groups was not statistically significant (Kumar et al. 2013). There have been reports of focal and generalized corneal edema, Descemet's membrane detachment, and even delayed corneal decompensation.

Anterior chamber bleeding is a common complication of LPI. Up to 36 % of patients develop this complication. Fortunately, it is often self-limiting and stops with gentle pressure on the eye applied with the contact lens (Jiang et al. 2012; Golan et al. 2013). If bleeding continues the iris vessel can be cauterized with the argon laser. The view may be compromised by the blood clot. The surgeon may wish to choose an alternative LPI site or wait for the blood to resolve, usually after 20–30 min. Anterior chamber bleeding can cause blurred vision for several days, elevation of IOP, and corneal endothelial blood staining. The risk of bleeding can be reduced by avoiding iris vessels and using pretreatment with argon laser (de Silva et al. 2012). Stopping antiplatelet therapy does not reduce the incidence of bleeding (Golan et al. 2013).

1.4.3.2   Postlaser Iridotomy Complications

The most common complication after LPI is postlaser IOP elevation, the incidence of which varies from 5.7 %–40 % depending on the definition of an IOP spike. A pressure spike usually occurs within the first 1 hour after LPI. The largest prospective study of primary angle closure suspects receiving LPI was from China. Of the 734 eyes, 9.8 % had an IOP spike of >8 mmHg, and only 0.54 % had an IOP >30 mmHg after 1 h. 0.82 % continued to have raised IOP at 2 weeks (Jiang et al. 2012). In another study that included both primary angle closure and angle closure suspects (therefore patients with angle pathology), the incidence of a postlaser IOP spike of more than 30 mmHg was higher at 7.2 % (Lee et al. 2014b). Some studies suggest that the energy used correlates to IOP spikes (Jiang et al. 2012), although other studies did not confirm this correlation (Lee et al. 2014b; Golan et al. 2013). A higher starting IOP is a risk factor for IOP spikes. Pre- and/or posttreatment with brimonidine 0.2 % or apraclonidine 0.5 % is helpful in preventing IOP spikes (Yuen et al. 2005). If the IOP is over 30 mmHg at 30–60 min after LPI medical management should be initiated. Topical beta blocker or oral acetazolamide can be considered. In rare cases, the IOP may not be controlled medically and filtration surgery may be required.

Mild iritis is a very common complication but usually resolves with topical steroids within a day. Cycloplegics are rarely required but posterior synechia may develop. In patients with active or known uveitis the inflammatory response from LPI can be severe. Intensive topical steroids and even systemic steroids may be necessary. Iridotomy closure may occur and repeated LPI attempts under steroid cover may be required.

Unusual visual symptoms have been reported following LPI such as diplopia, lines, shadows, or ghost images. Linear dysphotopsia is thought to be most specific to LPI. A Canadian study found that it occurs in around 6.8 % of eyes after LPI. A superior LPI is 3.6 times more likely to cause linear dysphotopsia than a temporally placed LPI (Vera et al. 2014). Partially or completely covered LPI by the eyelid was four times more likely to have these symptoms than an uncovered LPI. This is thought to be due to the prismatic effect of the tear film at the lid margin. However, a large, prospective Chinese study found visual acuity and retinal staylight measurements to be the same in both the LPI and the untreated control eye. They also found that subjective glare and visual symptoms did not differ significantly among those with LPI that were uncovered, partially covered, or completely covered. There was no association between size of LPI and glare symptoms (Congdon et al. 2012).

The difference in findings between the Chinese and Canadian studies may be cultural. Nevertheless, it is important to inform patients about this potential complication and to give patients time as many will adapt to this symptom. In the event that the patient is unable to tolerate the symptoms, an opaque contact lens or corneal tattooing can be considered. Other rare complications include retinal burns, macular hole, retinal detachment, choroidal effusion, malignant glaucoma, cataract formation, and zonular weakening.

Key Points
- Pretreatment with argon laser is helpful in dark iris patients to reduce risk of bleeding and pigment release.
- Iris bleeding can be stopped by applying pressure on the eye with the contact lens. Persistent bleeding can be cauterized using argon laser.
- Stopping antiplatelet therapy does not reduce the incidence of iris bleeding.
- Intraocular pressure spikes are common and alpha-agonist prophylaxis is helpful. Intraocular pressure should be checked 30–60 min after the procedure and managed accordingly.
- Iritis is common and topical steroids should be given to all patients.
- The iridotomy location should be uncovered by the eyelid to reduce the risk of dysphotopsia.

1.5   Lasers That Increase Angle Width: Argon Laser Iridoplasty

1.5.1   Introduction

Argon laser iridoplasty (ALP) is a procedure to open an appositionally closed angle. Laser peripheral iridotomy (LPI) is the definitive treatment for pupil block, but ALP can be helpful in other causes of angle closure such as plateau iris.

ALP can be useful in the acute setting when the cornea is cloudy, the anterior chamber is very shallow and the eye is inflamed. LPI may be difficult to perform in this setting and ALP can temporarily relieve the high IOP. Once the IOP is reduced, the cornea can clear, the eye is less inflamed, and the patient is more comfortable. All published data have reported a good success rate at breaking the acute attack (Ritch et al. 2007). At this point, the surgeon can decide to proceed with either LPI or lens extraction. Studies have shown that primary ALP is as effective as medical treatment in the management of acute angle closure glaucoma and acute phacomorphic glaucoma (Lam et al. 2002; Lee et al. 2013).

ALP may also be helpful for the management of chronic angle closure, plateau iris syndrome, nanophthalmos, peripheral anterior synechiae, lens related angle closure, and choroidal effusion-related angle closure. Recently, ALP has been reported to help reshape and realign the pupil centrally in decentered multifocal intraocular lenses. There are reports where this has improved distance and near vision (Solomon et al. 2012).

1.5.2   Procedure

ALP is performed under topical anesthesia in the outpatient setting. Pilocarpine 1–4 % is given three times over 10–30 min. Topical glycerin can be used in extreme cases to clear corneal edema in acute glaucoma if iris detail is not visible. Argon laser settings are 500 μm spot size, 0.5 s duration, and 200–400 MW power. An Abraham or Weiss iridotomy contact lens should be used. The aiming beam is focused on the peripheral iris close to the limbus. The aim is to create large contracting burns. The power should be reduced if there is any bubble formation or popping noises. The laser applications should be one to two spot sizes apart and never adjoining. Postoperative brimonidine 0.2 % or apraclonidine 0.5 % should be given immediately. The IOP should be checked 30–60 min after the procedure and posttreatment steroids given four to six times a day for 5–7 days.

1.5.3   Complications

Mild iritis is a common finding. The inflammation is usually transient and responds well to topical steroids. In severe cases, peripheral anterior synechiae, anterior chamber fibrin, or hypopyon can occur. In the inflamed eye or in known uveitic patients, the topical steroid strength and frequency should be increased to hourly for the first 2 days, with regular follow-up. Peri-orbital or systemic steroids can also be considered in extreme cases.

Post-ALP IOP spikes are not as common as after LPI. Postoperative brimonidine 0.2 % or apraclonidine 0.5 % is helpful. A study reported that only 1 out of 23 eyes had an IOP spike following ALP for plateau iris syndrome (Ritch et al. 2007). Raised IOP should be monitored closely and usually responds well to medical treatment.

Endothelial burns can occur in very shallow anterior chambers and in cases of poor visualization due to corneal edema. Care must be taken to focus on the iris. The surgeon can consider applying the laser in two concentric rings. The first ring is placed more centrally where the anterior chamber is deeper, to deepen the anterior chamber, followed by a second more peripheral ring of laser. In a flat anterior chamber or cases of extensive corneal edema or opacification, ALP is contraindicated. Burns from ALP are usually larger and more opaque compared to burns seen in iridotomy. The endothelial burns usually disappear in a few days (Ritch et al. 2007) but there have been reports of localized or general corneal edema and decompensation.

Iris atrophy and a nonreactive pupil can occur after ALP. A case series of 12 eyes in eight patients reported Urrets–Zavalia syndrome after ALP for persistent occludable angles after ALP. IOP increased in one eye. Seven patients had blurred vision, two had photophobia, four had glare, and one had discomfort. The mydriasis did not respond to pilocarpine, but resolved within 1 year (Espana et al. 2007). In patients receiving ALP for acute glaucoma, the incidence of iris atrophy and nonreactive pupil are much higher. Lai reported this complication in 8/33 eyes (24 %) at 3 years postlaser (Lai et al. 2002).

Pigmented burn marks may develop at the locations of laser applications and corectopia may occur, but are generally of no serious consequence (Lai et al. 2002). Patients may notice a change in the color of the peripheral iris or a distorted pupil and should be counseled accordingly.

Not all complications found after LPI occur following ALP. Iris hemorrhage does not occur in ALP due to the lower power density and the coagulative nature of argon laser. Lenticular opacification has not been reported.

1.6   Lasers That Reduce Aqueous Production: Transscleral Photocoagulation

1.6.1   Introduction

Transscleral laser photocoagulation was described by Beckman and Sugar in the early 1970s. Several types of lasers have been used including ruby laser and Nd:YAG laser and the technique has evolved from noncontact to contract with a fiber optic delivery probe. Transscleral diode cyclophotocoagulation (TCP) has become increasingly popular as it has good penetration and absorption by the pigmented tissue of the ciliary body.

1.6.2 Procedure

The procedure can be performed under a retrobulbar block or with general anesthesia. It can be performed using either an Nd:YAG or a diode laser. The Nd:YAG laser has a rounded sapphire probe tip that is placed 1–2 mm posterior to the limbus. Energy settings range from 4 to 9 W for 0.5–0.7 s.

For the 810-nm diode laser, energy levels start at 1500 mW with 2 s duration and are titrated to just below an audible "pop" sound, which indicates overtreatment. The number of applications is 17–20. The diode laser has a tip shaped as a footplate, where the heel is positioned at the limbus, so that treatment is delivered 1.2 mm posteriorly. The tip needs to be applied firmly to the eye to avoid conjunctival burns. The positioning of the laser probe may need to be altered in cases of a posterior ciliary body such as buphthalmos. Retroillumination of the globe can facilitate locating the ciliary body. Postoperative medications include atropine and steroid drops, in addition to continuing prelaser glaucoma medications.

1.6.3 Efficacy and Outcomes

Numerous studies have evaluated the efficacy of TCP. The response rate is 12.3–66 % with 54–92.7 % (average 73.7 %) obtaining an IOP of 21 mmHg or less after follow-up periods of 1–2 years (Ishida 2013). Some studies have found a correlation between a higher amount of energy delivered leading to a better pressure lowering effect (Hauber and Scherer 2002). However, this has not been observed in several other studies (Mistlberger et al. 2001). Factors that decrease the success rate include younger age, posttraumatic cases, and secondary glaucoma with previous vitreoretinal surgery. The outcome is typically less predictable than in other glaucoma surgeries, with rates of retreatment ranging from 20 to 40 % after 1 year.

1.6.4 Complications

1.6.4.1 Intraoperative Complications
Conjunctival burns can be produced if the probe is not placed firmly against the eye. Pupil ovalization or an atonic pupil can result. This risk may be decreased by avoiding the 3 and 9-o'clock positions. Hyphema or vitreous hemorrhage can occur, particularly in neovascular glaucoma.

1.6.4.2 Early Postoperative Complications
Patients may experience pain, photophobia and pigment dispersion. Rare complications described include lens subluxation, necrotizing scleritis and malignant glaucoma. Most patients experience a variable degree of anterior uveitis post-operatively that resolves with steroid treatment. A small subset of patients will develop persistent anterior chamber inflammation, due to disruption of the blood aqueous barrier. As this is not a true inflammatory reaction, these patients do not require long-term

steroid treatment. IOP fluctuations are common, and 10 % of patients will develop a significant IOP spike, particularly in those with neovascular glaucoma.

1.6.4.3   Late Postoperative Complications

The two main complications following TCP are hypotony (possibly leading to phthisis) and vision loss. Other late complications include cataract progression, chronic uveitis, cystoid macular edema and sympathetic ophthalmia (incidence of 0.07–0.7 %). The rate of corneal graft failure is 21 % (Tandon et al. 2014).

Hypotony occurs in 0–25 % of cases and phthisis in 0–9.9 % (Iliev and Gerber 2007). The risk of hypotony and phthisis is related to the amount of laser energy delivered. The lowest incidence of hypotony was seen in treatment protocols employing less than 80 J per treatment session. Independent risk factors for hypotony and phthisis are neovascular glaucoma, high pretreatment IOP, and uveitic glaucoma. For patients with primary open-angle glaucoma (POAG) these complication rates are lower (hypotony: 0–1.1 % and phthisis: 0–1.6 %). This is likely due to a lower pretreatment IOP, less energy delivered, and less advanced disease.

Loss of more than two Snellen lines occurs on average in 22.5 % of patients (range 0–55.2 %) (Ishida 2013). In a series by Schuman et al. (1992) of 116 eyes with advanced glaucoma treated with contact Nd:YAG TCP, 16 % progressed to no light perception and 47 % of eyes with a prelaser vision of 20/200 or better lost two or more Snellen lines. Hypotony was seen in 8 % (5 % had an IOP of 0). Another large series of 59 eyes followed up for a mean of 19 months (Spencer and Vernon 1999), reported that 32 % of patients with pretreatment vision better than 20/60 dropped two lines or more, and two patients with poor initial visual acuity dropped to no light perception. No factors have been predictive of vision loss after TCP, although patients with worse pretreatment vision tend to be at a higher risk of losing further vision. It is also unclear the extent that vision loss is due to the procedure versus the natural progression of the disease.

> **Key Points**
> - Patients should be counseled for pain and photophobia after the procedure and adequate anti-inflammatories and analgesia should be prescribed.
> - The risk of hypotony, vision loss, and phthisis is low if less than 80 J of energy is delivered per treatment session

1.7   Lasers That Reduce Aqueous Production: Endocyclophotocoagulation

1.7.1   Introduction

First described in 1992, a newer method to directly photocoagulate the ciliary processes under endoscopic guidance, known as endoscopic diode cyclophotocoagulation (ECP), is performed in conjunction with cataract or vitreoretinal surgery. It can be done in eyes with a good visual potential, but the pressure lowering effect is less compared to TCP.

1.7.2 Procedure

The laser probe (18-gauge or 20-gauge) can be inserted via a limbal or pars plana approach. It can be performed with a retrobulbar block or general anesthesia. When combined with cataract surgery, topical anesthesia with intracameral supplementation can be used, although a retrobulbar block is frequently employed. Energy is applied to each process until shrinkage and whitening occur (0.3–0.9 W), treating 270°–360°. If using a pars plana approach, a limited anterior vitrectomy is performed to allow adequate and safe access to the ciliary processes.

1.7.3 Efficacy and Outcomes

ECP is usually performed in two types of glaucoma, mild POAG or advanced secondary glaucoma. In a large series of patients with POAG, mean IOP decreased 7 mmHg (31 % decrease, range 3.9–10.9 mmHg decrease) after 2 years. In secondary glaucoma, the mean decrease was 50 % (range 26–68 %) (Kaplowitz et al. 2014) after a follow-up of 2–5 years. No factors that decrease the efficacy of treatment have been identified. However, poor results have been seen when used for congenital glaucoma, with a failure rate of 78 % at 5 years. The main problem with ECP is the frequent need for laser reapplications (probably due to regeneration of the ciliary epithelium). There is no long-term data on ECP, but it is suggested that success rates drop rapidly below 50 % after 36 months. A large retrospective study, however, found IOP under 21 mmHg in 79 % of patients after 5 years, on an average of 1.9 medications (Lima et al. 2010).

1.7.4 Complications

1.7.4.1 Intraoperative Complications
Complications including choroidal hemorrhages and retinal tears/detachment (1 %) can occur, particularly with the pars plana approach. Iris burns occur in 5 % of cases.

1.7.4.2 Early Postoperative Complications
The three most common early post-ECP complications are fibrin in the anterior chamber (7–22 %), hyphema (11 %), and CME (1–10 %) (Chen et al. 1997). Fibrinous uveitis usually responds to topical steroids and resolves in 4–10 weeks. Hyphema clears with conservative measures but may require surgical intervention. An IOP spike is seen in 10–14.4 % of patients. Endophthalmitis is a complication of any intraocular surgery, but the incidence following ECP is unknown. Corneal edema occurs in 4 % of cases and corneal graft failure in 8 %.

1.7.4.3 Late Postoperative Complications

Hypotony can occur in up to 18 % of cases. Larger retrospective studies have reported hypotony rates ranging from 1.2 to 9 % (Lima et al. 2010; Murthy et al. 2009) after 2–5 years. The endoscope can be used to look for changes in the ciliary processes and to perform a fibrous membrane dissection, which has been shown to increase IOP. Phthisis can occur in up to 2.5 % of patients (Lima et al. 2004). Incidence of vision loss of more than two lines has been described in 1–6 % (Chen et al. 1997) in studies that have 2–5 years of follow-up. Loss of vision seems to be related to the severity of the glaucoma, with up to 24 % of patients with advanced glaucoma losing vision. Cataract progression occurs in 24.5 % of patients. CME has been reported to occur in 0.7–10 %. To date no cases of sympathetic ophthalmia have been reported following ECP.

References

Barkana Y, Belkin M. Selective laser trabeculoplasty. Surv Ophthalmol. 2007;52(6):634–54. doi:10.1016/j.survophthal.2007.08.014.

Chen J, Cohn RA, Lin SC, Cortes AE, Alvarado JA. Endoscopic photocoagulation of the ciliary body for treatment of refractory glaucomas. Am J Ophthalmol. 1997;124(6):787–96.

Coakes R. Laser trabeculoplasty. Br J Ophthalmol. 1992;76(10):624–6.

Congdon N, Yan X, Friedman DS, Foster PJ, van den Berg TJ, Peng M, Gangwani R, He M. Visual symptoms and retinal straylight after laser peripheral iridotomy: the Zhongshan Angle-Closure Prevention Trial. Ophthalmology. 2012;119(7):1375–82. doi:10.1016/j.ophtha.2012.01.015.

Damji KF, Bovell AM, Hodge WG, Rock W, Shah K, Buhrmann R, Pan YI. Selective laser trabeculoplasty versus argon laser trabeculoplasty: results from a 1-year randomised clinical trial. Br J Ophthalmol. 2006;90(12):1490–4. doi:10.1136/bjo.2006.098855.

de Silva DJ, Day AC, Bunce C, Gazzard G, Foster PJ. Randomised trial of sequential pretreatment for Nd:YAG laser iridotomy in dark irides. Br J Ophthalmol. 2012;96(2):263–6. doi:10.1136/bjo.2010.200030.

de Silva DJ, Gazzard G, Foster P. Laser iridotomy in dark irides. Br J Ophthalmol. 2007;91(2):222–5. doi:10.1136/bjo.2006.104315.

Espana EM, Ioannidis A, Tello C, Liebmann JM, Foster P, Ritch R. Urrets-Zavalia syndrome as a complication of argon laser peripheral iridoplasty. Br J Ophthalmol. 2007;91(4):427–9. doi:10.1136/bjo.2006.105098.

Fea AM, Bosone A, Rolle T, Brogliatti B, Grignolo FM. Micropulse diode laser trabeculoplasty (MDLT): a phase II clinical study with 12 months follow-up. Clin Ophthalmol. 2008;2(2):247–52.

Fleck BW. How large must an iridotomy be? Br J Ophthalmol. 1990;74(10):583–8.

Fudemberg SJ, Myers JS, Katz LJ. Trabecular meshwork tissue examination with scanning electron microscopy: a comparison of micropulse diode laser (MLT), selective laser (SLT), and argon laser (ALT) trabeculoplasty in human cadaver tissue. Invest Ophthalmol Vis Sci. 2008;49(5):1236.

Glaucoma laser trial. Ophthalmology. 1991;98(6):841–3.

Golan S, Levkovitch-Verbin H, Shemesh G, Kurtz S. Anterior chamber bleeding after laser peripheral iridotomy. JAMA Ophthalmol. 2013;131(5):626–9. doi:10.1001/jamaophthalmol.2013.1642.

Goldenfeld M, Melamed S, Simon G, Ben Simon GJ. Titanium:sapphire laser trabeculoplasty versus argon laser trabeculoplasty in patients with open-angle glaucoma. Ophthalmic Surg Lasers Imaging. 2009;40(3):264–9.

Gossage D. Two-year data on MicroPulse laser trabeculoplasty. 2015. Eye world. Retried from URL: http://www.eyeworld.org/article-two-year-data-on-micropulse-laser-trabeculoplasty. Accessed on 1 June 2015.

Hauber FA, Scherer WJ. Influence of total energy delivery on success rate after contact diode laser transscleral cyclophotocoagulation: a retrospective case review and meta-analysis. J Glaucoma. 2002;11(4):329–33.

Iliev ME, Gerber S. Long-term outcome of trans-scleral diode laser cyclophotocoagulation in refractory glaucoma. Br J Ophthalmol. 2007;91(12):1631–5. doi:10.1136/bjo.2007.116533.

Ishida K. Update on results and complications of cyclophotocoagulation. Curr Opin Ophthalmol. 2013;24(2):102–10. doi:10.1097/ICU.0b013e32835d9335.

Jiang Y, Chang DS, Foster PJ, He M, Huang S, Aung T, Friedman DS. Immediate changes in intraocular pressure after laser peripheral iridotomy in primary angle-closure suspects. Ophthalmology. 2012;119(2):283–8. doi:10.1016/j.ophtha.2011.08.014.

Jinapriya D, D'Souza M, Hollands H, El-Defrawy SR, Irrcher I, Smallman D, Farmer JP, Cheung J, Urton T, Day A, Sun X, Campbell RJ. Anti-inflammatory therapy after selective laser trabeculoplasty: a randomized, double-masked, placebo-controlled clinical trial. Ophthalmology. 2014;121(12):2356–61. doi:10.1016/j.ophtha.2014.07.017.

Juhas T. Sympathetic ophthalmia as a complication of argon laser trabeculoplasty. Ocul Immunol Inflamm. 1993;1(1–2):67–70. doi:10.3109/09273949309086540.

Kaplowitz K, Kuei A, Klenofsky B, Abazari A, Honkanen R. The use of endoscopic cyclophotocoagulation for moderate to advanced glaucoma. Acta Ophthalmol. 2014; doi:10.1111/aos.12529.

Klamann MK, Maier AK, Gonnermann J, Ruokonen PC. Adverse effects and short-term results after selective laser trabeculoplasty. J Glaucoma. 2014;23(2):105–8. doi:10.1097/IJG.0b013e3182684fd1.

Knickelbein JE, Singh A, Flowers BE, Nair UK, Eisenberg M, Davis R, Raju LV, Schuman JS, Conner IP. Acute corneal edema with subsequent thinning and hyperopic shift following selective laser trabeculoplasty. J Cataract Refract Surg. 2014;40(10):1731–5. doi:10.1016/j.jcrs.2014.08.002.

Koucheki B, Hashemi H. Selective laser trabeculoplasty in the treatment of open-angle glaucoma. J Glaucoma. 2012;21(1):65–70. doi:10.1097/IJG.0b013e3182027596.

Kumar RS, Baskaran M, Friedman DS, Xu Y, Wong HT, Lavanya R, Chew PT, Foster PJ, Aung T. Effect of prophylactic laser iridotomy on corneal endothelial cell density over 3 years in primary angle closure suspects. Br J Ophthalmol. 2013;97(3):258–61. doi:10.1136/bjophthalmol-2012-302013.

Lai JS, Tham CC, Chua JK, Poon AS, Lam DS. Laser peripheral iridoplasty as initial treatment of acute attack of primary angle-closure: a long-term follow-up study. J Glaucoma. 2002;11(6):484–7.

Lam DS, Lai JS, Tham CC, Chua JK, Poon AS. Argon laser peripheral iridoplasty versus conventional systemic medical therapy in treatment of acute primary angle-closure glaucoma: a prospective, randomized, controlled trial. Ophthalmology. 2002;109(9):1591–6.

Lee JW, Chan JC, Chang RT, Singh K, Liu CC, Gangwani R, Wong MO, Lai JS. Corneal changes after a single session of selective laser trabeculoplasty for open-angle glaucoma. Eye (Lond). 2014a;28(1):47–52. doi:10.1038/eye.2013.231.

Lee JW, Lai JS, Yick DW, Yuen CY. Argon laser peripheral iridoplasty versus systemic intraocular pressure-lowering medications as immediate management for acute phacomorphic angle closure. Clin Ophthalmol. 2013;7:63–9. doi:10.2147/OPTH.S39503.

Lee JW, Wong MO, Liu CC, Lai JS. Optimal selective laser trabeculoplasty energy for maximal intraocular pressure reduction in open-angle glaucoma. J Glaucoma. 2015; doi:10.1097/IJG.0000000000000215.

Lee TL, Yuxin Ng J, Nongpiur ME, Tan WJ, Aung T, Perera SA. Intraocular pressure spikes after a sequential laser peripheral iridotomy for angle closure. J Glaucoma. 2014b;23(9):644–8. doi:10.1097/IJG.0b013e318285fdaa.

Lima FE, Carvalho DM, Avila MP. Phacoemulsification and endoscopic cyclophotocoagulation as primary surgical procedure in coexisting cataract and glaucoma. Arq Bras Oftalmol. 2010;73(5):419–22.

Lima FE, Magacho L, Carvalho DM, Susanna Jr R, Avila MP. A prospective, comparative study between endoscopic cyclophotocoagulation and the Ahmed drainage implant in refractory glaucoma. J Glaucoma. 2004;13(3):233–7.

Mistlberger A, Liebmann JM, Tschiderer H, Ritch R, Ruckhofer J, Grabner G. Diode laser transscleral cyclophotocoagulation for refractory glaucoma. J Glaucoma. 2001;10(4):288–93.

Moubayed SP, Hamid M, Choremis J, Li G. An unusual finding of corneal edema complicating selective laser trabeculoplasty. Can J Ophthalmol. 2009;44(3):337–8. doi:10.3129/i09-025.

Murthy GJ, Murthy PR, Murthy KR, Kulkarni VV, Murthy KR. A study of the efficacy of endoscopic cyclophotocoagulation for the treatment of refractory glaucomas. Indian J Ophthalmol. 2009;57(2):127–32.

Narayanaswamy A, Leung CK, Istiantoro DV, Perera SA, Ho CL, Nongpiur ME, Baskaran M, Htoon HM, Wong TT, Goh D, Su DH, Belkin M, Aung T. Efficacy of selective laser trabeculoplasty in primary angle-closure glaucoma: a randomized clinical trial. JAMA Ophthalmol. 2014; doi:10.1001/jamaophthalmol.2014.4893.

Ong K, Ong L. Selective laser trabeculoplasty may compromise corneas with pigment on endothelium. Clin Experiment Ophthalmol. 2013;41(1):109–110; question and answer 111–2. doi:10.1111/j.1442-9071.2012.02841.x

Ritch R, Tham CC, Lam DS. Argon laser peripheral iridoplasty (ALPI): an update. Surv Ophthalmol. 2007;52(3):279–88. doi:10.1016/j.survophthal.2007.02.006.

Schuman JS, Bellows AR, Shingleton BJ, Latina MA, Allingham RR, Belcher CD, Puliafito CA. Contact transscleral Nd:YAG laser cyclophotocoagulation. Midterm results. Ophthalmology. 1992;99(7):1089–1094; discussion 1095.

Silver DM, Quigley HA. Aqueous flow through the iris-lens channel: estimates of differential pressure between the anterior and posterior chambers. J Glaucoma. 2004;13(2):100–7.

Solomon R, Barsam A, Voldman A, Holladay J, Bhogal M, Perry HD, Donnenfeld ED. Argon laser iridoplasty to improve visual function following multifocal intraocular lens implantation. J Refract Surg. 2012;28(4):281–3. doi:10.3928/1081597X-20120209-01.

Spencer AF, Vernon SA. "Cyclodiode": results of a standard protocol. Br J Ophthalmol. 1999;83(3):311–6.

Stein JD, Challa P. Mechanisms of action and efficacy of argon laser trabeculoplasty and selective laser trabeculoplasty. Curr Opin Ophthalmol. 2007;18(2):140–5. doi:10.1097/ICU.0b013e328086aebf.

Tandon A, Espandar L, Cupp D, Ho S, Johnson V, Ayyala RS. Surgical management for postkeratoplasty glaucoma: a meta-analysis. J Glaucoma. 2014;23(7):424–9. doi:10.1097/IJG.0b013e31827a0712.

Vera V, Naqi A, Belovay GW, Varma DK, Ahmed II. Dysphotopsia after temporal versus superior laser peripheral iridotomy: a prospective randomized paired eye trial. Am J Ophthalmol. 2014;157(5):929–35. doi:10.1016/j.ajo.2014.02.010.

Weinreb RN, Wilensky JT. Clinical aspects of argon laser trabeculoplasty. Int Ophthalmol Clin. 1984;24(3):79–95.

Wong MO, Lee JW, Choy BN, Chan JC, Lai JS. Systematic review and meta-analysis on the efficacy of selective laser trabeculoplasty in open-angle glaucoma. Surv Ophthalmol. 2015;60(1):36–50. doi:10.1016/j.survophthal.2014.06.006.

Yuen NS, Cheung P, Hui SP. Comparing brimonidine 0.2 % to apraclonidine 1.0 % in the prevention of intraocular pressure elevation and their pupillary effects following laser peripheral iridotomy. Jpn J Ophthalmol. 2005;49(2):89–92. doi:10.1007/s10384-004-0149-9.

Kuang Hu, Keith Barton, and Julian Garcia Feijoo

2.1 Introduction

Minimally invasive glaucoma surgery (MIGS) interventions are intended to deliver reduction of intraocular pressure (IOP) with a better safety profile than conventional glaucoma surgery. There has been active development of novel MIGS devices and implants, and these continue to evolve.

The role of MIGS is the subject of some uncertainty. Although it is generally accepted that MIGS interventions are not as effective as conventional glaucoma drainage surgery, their better safety profiles may make them suitable for patients who do not require very low intraocular pressures to control their glaucoma. To resolve such debates, high-quality randomized controlled trial data are required. When MIGS is being combined with cataract surgery, trials need to disentangle the effect of phacoemulsification from that of MIGS because phacoemulsification itself is known to lower intraocular pressure (Chen et al. 2015; Mansberger et al. 2012). Moreover, the role of MIGS may not be fully established by studies that focus solely on efficacy and safety. Rather, patients' quality of life and cost-effectiveness in comparison to conventional medical and surgical treatments need to be taken into account.

Presently, MIGS techniques are designed to increase the outflow of aqueous in one of several ways. External drainage devices such as the XEN Gel Implant permit drainage of aqueous into the subconjunctival space. Trabecular bypass techniques

K. Hu (✉)
Moorfields Eye Hospital NHS Foundation Trust, London, UK
e-mail: kuanghu@kuanghu.com

K. Barton
Glaucoma Service, Moorfields Eye Hospital, 162 City Road, London EC1V 2PD, UK

J.G. Feijoo
Department of Ophthalmology, Hospital Clinico San Carlos, Universidad Complutense, Instituto de Investigacion Sanitaria HCSC, OFTARED, Madrid, Spain

F. Carbonaro, K. Sheng Lim (eds.), *Managing Complications in Glaucoma Surgery*,
DOI 10.1007/978-3-319-49416-6_2, © Springer International Publishing AG 2017

such as iStent, Trabectome, and Hydrus aim to improve access of aqueous from the anterior chamber to Schlemm's canal and thence to functional collector channels. Choroidal shunts such as CyPass are designed to increase drainage of aqueous into the suprachoroidal space. This chapter will focus on the devices mentioned above. The principles that emerge are likely to be applicable to other MIGS techniques, both current and future.

2.2   Trans-trabecular Meshwork Surgeries

2.2.1   iStent

2.2.1.1   Safety and Efficacy

Randomized controlled trials on the first-generation version of the iStent (Glaukos, Laguna Hills, USA) focused on its use with concomitant phacoemulsification (Craven et al. 2012; Fea 2010; Samuelson et al. 2011).

In an industry-funded open-label trial involving 240 patients with open-angle glaucoma controlled with topical medications, implantation of iStent in conjunction with cataract surgery was compared to cataract surgery alone (Samuelson et al. 2011). Seventy-two percent of eyes treated with iStent versus 50 % of control eyes achieved IOP of 21 mmHg or lower without use of medication at 12 months. Stent obstruction was observed in 4 % of subjects and 4 % required stent-related secondary surgery in the form of repositioning or replacement. At 15 months postoperatively in a separate double-masked randomized controlled trial (Fea 2010), 67 % of eyes with primary open-angle glaucoma having iStent implantation at the time of cataract surgery did not require topical medication versus 24 % of eyes who had cataract surgery alone. At 24 months, patients with stents appear to be more likely than those without to achieve IOP of 21 mmHg or lower without medication, though there was no overall difference in ocular hypotensive medication between the two groups (Craven et al. 2012).

A second generation of device, called the iStent inject, has been developed. This has a conical shape and is provided on an injector preloaded with two devices.

In a prospective unmasked study (Voskanyan et al. 2014), two iStent inject devices were implanted in each of 99 patients who had open-angle glaucoma that was uncontrolled on two or more topical medications. Two-thirds of subjects achieved an IOP of 18 mmHg or lower without medication at 12 months. The commonest postoperative complications were elevated IOP (10 %) and stent obstruction (3 %). Secondary surgery was performed in 3 % of patients for elevated IOP. The stent was not visible gonioscopically in 13 % of patients.

An industry-sponsored prospective unmasked randomized trial enrolling 192 subjects (Fea et al. 2014) found that implantation of two iStent inject devices was at least as effective in terms of IOP control as medical therapy with the fixed combination of latanoprost and timolol (Xalacom, Pfizer) in patients who had open-angle glaucoma that was not controlled with a single topical medication. At 12 months, 95 % of eyes treated with stents and 92 % of eyes treated with Xalacom achieved

IOP reduction of at least 20 %. 93% of eyes achieved IOP of less than or equal to 18 mmHg in the stent group versus 90 % of eyes in the Xalacom group. One of the 94 patients in the stent group experienced "decompensation" of IOP to 48 mmHg.

2.2.1.2 Procedure

IStent surgery can be performed under topical anesthesia and intracameral anesthesia is recommended. The trabecular stent can be implanted through the clear corneal incision used for phacoemulsification in cases of combined surgery or through a 1.5 mm incision when the stent is implanted as an isolated operation. A wider incision facilitates surgical maneuvers and is recommended during the learning curve, as this facilitates a better implantation angle especially when more than one implantation attempt is required. The injection of acetylcholine into the anterior chamber is advisable in phakic patients as this minimizes risk of lens damage. In the majority of cases, the corneal incision should be temporal so allowing the stent to be implanted in the nasal region of the trabecular meshwork, where the number of collecting channels is greatest.

The G1 Glaukos® trabecular micro-bypass (GT100) is made of titanium and covered with a layer of heparin (Duraflo® powder). It is L-shaped, measures 1×0.4 mm with an external diameter of 180 μm and is designed to fit within the lumen of the canal. The end of the canal portion is pointed to allow penetration through the meshwork during insertion. Three retention ridges spaced along the half-pipe portion allow for secure placement of the micro-bypass. The stent is preloaded in a 26-gauge insertion device with a release button. The stent is usually implanted through a temporal approach in a nasal position. If two implants are used, one is placed inferonasally and the other superonasally.

Before starting the iStent procedure, the head of the patient must be repositioned at 45° to the opposite side of the eye undergoing surgery, while tilting the microscope 30° for a good view of the trabecular meshwork on the nasal side of the angle using a Swan–Jacob gonioscope. After filling the anterior chamber with viscoelastic and checking the visualization of the angle, the inserter is introduced into the anterior chamber. The tip of the iStent should approach the trabecular meshwork at an angle of 15° to facilitate penetration. The point of the trabecular micro-bypass must go through the trabecular meshwork and softly advance through the Schlemm's canal. Once the trabecular meshwork covers all of the implant, it is released by pressing the applicator button. Only the proximal end of the stent should remain visible in the anterior chamber. The stent can be seated in its final position by gently tapping the side of the snorkel with the inserter tip. The stent should be placed parallel to the plane of the iris with the inner part covered by the meshwork and the lumen away from the iris. A small reflux of blood from the Schlemm's canal is common and reflects adequate positioning of the stent. Excessive resistance indicates a path that is too perpendicular to the trabeculum. If difficulty is encountered with insertion at the primary location, it is recommended finding another location inferiorly or superiorly or try inserting 0.5 clock hours inferiorly, and continue to move inferiorly as needed for subsequent attempts. At the end of the procedure, the anterior chamber is flushed to eliminate any refluxed blood. This ensures good visualization to confirm that the implant is well located at sufficient depth. The viscoelastic agent can then be removed and the anterior chamber filled with saline solution.

In combined surgery the same corneal incision can be used. When phacoemulsification has been completed acetylcholine can be injected, then the anterior chamber should be refilled with a cohesive viscoelastic and then proceed as previously described.

For iStent inject (GTS400) the procedure is similar. This implant is conic and smaller than the G1 and also made of titanium. The Stents are preloaded in the customized injector system designed to deliver the stents automatically into the Schlemm's canal. To do so the inserter should be positioned in the desired position in contact with the angle but not pushing the tissue. The injector features a release button on the housing so by pressing this button the stent is released into the Schlemm's canal.

2.2.1.3 Patient Selection and Indications

The best indications for the trabecular stent are cases with primary open-angle, pigmentary, or pseudoexfoliative glaucoma. In secondary open-angle glaucoma, this type of surgery may be indicated as long as the Schlemm's canal and collecting channels are found to be undamaged. A good indication is corticosteroid-induced glaucoma (Morales-Fernandez et al. 2012). The ideal candidate for this type of surgery is a patient with early or moderate stage glaucoma, also patients with compliance issues, low tolerance to medical treatment or simply patients reluctant to undergo a chronic daily treatment. Another indication could be high-risk OHT or early/mid-disease patients with high IOP or suboptimal IOP control but in which a conventional filtering surgery may be too aggressive.

Patients with advanced glaucoma or those who require very low target pressures to obtain stabilization of their disease are not suitable candidates. Nevertheless, iStent could be considered in some cases when a filtering procedure is not recommended or refused by the patient.

Candidates for combined surgery using the iStent are patients with cataract and open-angle glaucoma with early/mild disease, even if they are well controlled on two or three medications.

2.2.1.4 Complications

The published evidence shows that, when performed with care iStent implantation is safe and the complication rate is very low. Visualization and correct selection of the area of implantation are key for a successful and effective implantation.

Selecting the Area of Implantation Preoperative evaluation of the areas with more collector channels is difficult. However, with the decompression of the anterior chamber the blood reflux can help identify the areas with more blood reflux. This is an indirect sign to determine the areas with more favorable anatomy and is especially helpful when the blood column is fragmented. If these areas are not accessible through the initial incision, the surgeon should consider making a new incision.

Intraoperative Complications
Prevention of Complications. Angle Visualization The most common mistake when performing the surgery the first few times is failure to position the microscope and/or the patient adequately in order to obtain an adequate view of the trabeculum. This step is crucial for all the angular surgeries described in this chapter, and the surgeon should take some time to assure the correct visualization and identification of the angular structures. This is more difficult when trabecular meshwork pigmentation is poor. So before introducing the inserter in the anterior chamber the surgeon should check the positions of the patient's head and the microscope together with the angle visualization. If visualization is not good enough, position should be adjusted. By following these steps, most of the complications related to the insertion procedure can be minimized.

Incorrect Implantation. iStent Position The implant should be completely inserted in the Schlemms's canal as described above, so the iStent final position should be parallel to the iris root with the ridges located on the back wall of Schlemm's canal. If it is too superficial or not completely introduced, it may fall out. Implantation angle is important and iStent position must be checked before it is released from the applicator. If the implant is not completely introduced the inserter tip can be used to tap the iStent into place. If snagged in the tissue or the iStent is outside the canal, or even if it was released before firmly anchored in place and is loose in the anterior chamber, it can be recovered with the inserter or retinal forceps. Then it is possible to reload the iStent onto the inserter and try again. In the series by Arriola-Villalobos et al. (2012), in 33.3 % of cases two attempts were required to implant the iStent correctly, and in 6 % of the cases a third attempt was needed.

Trabecular Meshwork Tear Once the implant is correctly positioned inside the Schlemm's canal, the surgeon must cease all movement and release the implant. If the movement continues once the iStent is inside the Schlemm's canal, the iStent tip will tear the trabecular meshwork. While this might be considered a minor complication, it will increase the trauma to the outer wall of the canal and even damage the collector channels. Moreover, with the loosening of the trabecular meshwork inner wall the tissue required to support the implant is lost. This consideration is also important if more than one attempt is needed. If during successive implantation attempts, an adequate implantation angle is not obtainable using the initial incision a new corneal incision could be performed if necessary.

Cyclodialysis Cleft. Suprachoroidal Implantation If the implantation technique is inadequate or, more frequently, visualization of the angle structures poor, then there is a risk of tearing the iris root with the iStent tip and inserting the iStent in the ciliary band or even introducing the implant in the supraciliary/suprachoroidal space. This risk is higher when several attempts are required and blood prevents adequate angle visualization. This increases the risk of bleeding that could also be more severe than usual. If the tear is limited and bleeding is not important the surgery can usually be completed. If the tear is longer and associated with a visible cleft or the bleeding becomes severe, the procedure should be cancelled.

If the angle structures are incorrectly identified and the ciliary band misidentified as the pigmented meshwork or if for any reason visualization is not good enough, there is a risk of implanting the device in the ciliary band or even deeper into the supraciliary/suprachoidal space. Even if intracameral anesthesia is used if the iStent touches the ciliary tissue or the iris root, the patient will feel some pain, so this is an important sign to recognize. In this case, the recommendation is to check the angle structures and positioning to be sure that the area of implantation has been correctly identified.

Iridectomy/Iridodialysis/Lens Damage Incorrect manipulation of the inserter in the anterior chamber may cause iris damage and even iridodialysis. This may also happen if the angle structures are not correctly identified or if the iris is caught on the tip of the iStent and the surgeon keeps moving the inserter. Moreover, these cases usually involve severe bleeding and this can make surgery more difficult. In phakic patients the surgeon may damage the lens with the inserter and even tear the anterior capsule of lens. To avoid this complication the use of acetylcholine is recommended in phakic eyes. Also introduce the inserter slightly up until the pupil is crossed instead of aiming directly at the angle.

Bleeding Some bleeding is common and usually indicates the blood reflux through the iStent. But it could be important in case of the complications described above. Ensuring a correct visualization of the angle is crucial. Also surgery should be carried out with gentle movements. In case of bleeding that prevents visualization the surgeon should wait until the bleeding decreases or stops completely. Then proceed to clean the anterior chamber and start the surgical procedure again. If bleeding is severe or visualization is not good enough the surgeon may have to consider cancelling or postponing the procedure.

Early Postoperative Complications

Malposition. Free Implant As mentioned above, it is important to verify the final implant position before the end of the surgery. If visualization was not good enough, it is important to check for the implant position postoperatively. If only the proximal part of the snorkel is outside the canal, no further intervention is usually needed and this will not interfere with the efficacy of the procedure. However, if it is just puncturing the tissue, outside the canal or positioned unattached in the angle or on the iris, the surgeon has to consider repositioning the implant to avoid possible future complications (and for the implant to be functional). However, even if the stents are detached from the trabecular meshwork they usually will settle on the angle and will not move (Arriola-Villalobos et al. 2012), since they are highly biocompatible and well tolerated they may also be left in the anterior chamber. In this case, adequate follow-up is needed and if inflammation or other problems are detected they should be removed (Fig. 2.1).

Fig. 2.1 Two malpositioned iStent implants

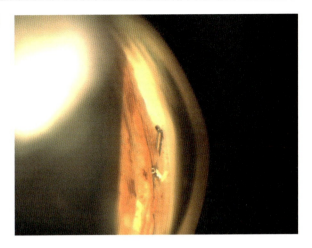

Superficial Implantation If the iStent is too superficial or incompletely inserted, there is a risk of detachment. In the case of superficial implantation, the iStent does not penetrate the trabecular meshwork completely and can be just engaged in the superficial layers of the trabecular meshwork. In this case there would be no communication between the anterior chamber and the Schlemm's canal so the implant would not be efficacious. Moreover, it could come loose over time. Repositioning should be considered, but as mentioned before, most of the time the implant will settle on the iris root and cause no problems.

Cyclodialysis Cleft/Suprachoroidal Implantation If IOP is very low during the first week a cyclodialysis cleft has to be ruled out. Also if the iStent is not seen in the angle and the iris root/ciliary tissue appear to have been damaged the area should be imaged with OCT or UBM to find the stent. Most of the cases can be managed conservatively as the cleft will close over time. If pressure remains too low or maculopathy develops, it may be necessary to suture the cleft. If the iStent is in the suprachoidal space but there is no inflammation removal is not necessary but close follow-up is required.

Late Postoperative Complications
A 5-year case series study by Arriola et al. showed no major complications regarding stent placement in the meshwork in a 19 patient study after 5 years (Arriola-Villalobos et al. 2012).

IStent obstruction If the Stent is rotated toward the iris, the anterior chamber is narrow and not very deep or the iris is floppy, the aqueous humor flow to the iStent could facilitate the blockage of the device with the iris. This situation can be resolved by lasering the iris in order to unblock the stent snorkel. This has been described for both implant types (Fernandez-Barrientos et al. 2010; Arriola-Villalobos et al. 2012; Arriola-Villalobos et al. 2013; Fea 2010; Samuelson et al. 2011).

Endothelial damage Arriola-Villalobos et al. (2013) analyzed prospectively the endothelial changes after combined surgery (Phaco + GTS400/Glaukos inject). At 2 years of follow-up the endothelial cell count decrease was 13.22 %, a reduction similar to that reported after phacoemulsification alone. However, if the implant was malpositioned and in contact with the corneal endothelium, it should be removed to avoid progressive endothelial damage.

2.2.2 Hydrus

2.2.2.1 Safety and Efficacy

The Hydrus Microstent (Ivantis, Irvine, USA) has been evaluated in an industry-funded randomized controlled trial in which 100 patients with open-angle glaucoma and cataract were randomized to receive either Hydrus implantation with concomitant phacoemulsification or phacoemulsification alone (Pfeiffer et al. 2015). Washed-out diurnal IOP was evaluated at baseline, 12 months and 24 months. IOP-lowering medications were allowed at other times if follow-up IOP exceeded 19 mmHg or there was evidence of progressive optic nerve damage or visual field loss. Mean diurnal IOP was calculated from measurements made using a two-person system (observer and reader), with at least two readings being made at each of three time points, spaced 4 h apart between 8 am and 4 pm.

At 24 months, the proportion of patients with 20 % reduction in washed-out diurnal IOP was 80 % in the treatment group compared to 46 % in the control group ($p = 0.0008$) assessed on an intention-to-treat basis. In a separate analysis that excluded patients who did not wash out medications for safety reasons, a 20 % reduction in washed-out diurnal IOP was achieved in 89 % of the treatment group versus 64 % of the control group ($p = 0.0140$). Washed-out mean diurnal IOP at 12 months was 16.6 mmHg in the treatment group versus 17.4 mmHg in the control group. At 24 months, washed-out mean diurnal IOP was 16.9 mmHg in the treatment group compared to 19.2 mmHg in the control group ($p = 0.0093$). The proportion of patients using no hypotensive medication at 24 months was 73 % in the treatment group compared to 38 % in the control group ($p = 0.0008$).

In terms of adverse events, peripheral anterior synechiae formation was noted in 19 % of treated patients versus 2 % of controls at 24 months ($p = 0.0077$). However, the presence of PAS was not thought to affect IOP or medication outcomes. Best-corrected visual acuity decreased by 2 lines in 2 patients in the treatment group, but resolved by 1 month. By month 3, best-corrected visual acuity was 20/40 or better in 96 % of subjects in the treatment group versus 90 % in the control group. Hypotony and stent migration were not found in the treatment group. Secondary glaucoma surgery was required in 2 % of the treatment group versus 4 % of the control group, and the difference was not statistically significant.

2.2.2.2 Patient Selection and Procedure

The Hydrus implant is an 8 mm crescent-shaped implantable device. The implant is very flexible, made from nitinol (a nickel/titanium alloy), and is preloaded onto a handheld delivery system. The device not only bypasses the trabecular meshwork but scaffolds and dilates the Schlemm's canal. Due to its flexibility it easily sits in the Schlemm's canal and dilates it. As it scaffolds around one quarter of the canal it can provide access to multiple aqueous channels.

The surgery set-up is similar to the IStent surgical procedure described above, and a goniolens is needed to visualize the angle. Surgery can be performed under topical anesthesia or the technique of choice of the surgeon. Acetylcholine can be used in combined procedures; it can be implanted through the same corneal incision used for the phacoemulsification. For Hydrus alone procedures the implant can be inserted through a 1–1.5 mm corneal incision. If the target implantation site is not easily accessible/visible through the phaco incision, a secondary incision can be performed opposite to the desired implantation site.

After filling the anterior chamber with viscoelastic the delivery system is introduced in the anterior chamber and advanced until the inserter tip comes into contact with the trabecular meshwork. The trabecular meshwork is perforated using the beveled tip of the cannula. Once opened the device is implanted into the Schlemm's canal by rotating the advancement mechanism with one finger. The inserter terminal segment should be positioned parallel to the canal (flat angle) and with the bevel pointing slightly up. Otherwise, during the delivery the device could move down and out of the canal. Also if the angle between the angular surface and the inserter is excessive or the position is forced there could be problems with the delivery. The implant should advance with little or no resistance, if resistance is found the implant can be retracted and the position can be cautiously modified.

Once the implant is in place, the central core wire of the delivery system is retracted, allowing the complete detachment of the implant. The inlet segment (1–2 mm) should remain in the anterior chamber and the rest of the implant in the canal. On confirmation of the implant position, surgery is completed once the viscoelastic has been removed.

Conceptually the indications of the Hydrus implant are similar to the iStent. But, due to the dual action of the Hydrus implant, which bypasses the trabecular meshwork and expands the Schlemm's canal thus giving access to multiple collector channels, it is possible that the IOP reduction could be higher than after iStent implantation. However, this higher efficacy has still to be established.

2.2.2.3 Complications

Reported complication rate is very low, and when performed in combination with phacoemulsification the rate is similar to a cataract alone procedure (Pfeiffer et al. 2015).

Intraoperative Complications

To avoid intraoperative complications it is very important to visualize the tip of the inserter, be careful when crossing the pupil with the inserter in phakic eyes and avoid any movement during the "injection" of the Hydrus into the Schlemm's canal. The inserter has to be held steady and kept in contact with the angular tissue with the bevel slightly up. Also, note that the rotation knob of the inserter can be adjusted so the position of the bevel is comfortable for the surgeon.

Bleeding When the procedure is performed correctly some bleeding is very common and also indicates the reflux of blood from the venous system. This bleeding will not affect the patient's recovery or the final outcome. The presence of blood in the Schlemm's canal can also help to detect the best areas for implantation. If when touching the trabecular meshwork the blood prevents the correct visualization of the tip or the progression of the device it may be necessary to retrieve the implant, wash out the blood and viscoelastic, wait for the bleeding to stop, and then proceed again with the implantation. If the device touches/ruptures the iris or is implanted in the ciliary body, the bleeding could be more severe and may take some time to stop. If visualization is not good and the surgeon is unsure of a possible damage to the iris or ciliary body, cancelling the procedure should be considered and then wait for the eye to recover.

Incomplete/incorrect insertion The implant should be inserted so that only the inlet is outside the canal. The insertion angle is extremely important and after opening the meshwork the bevel should be angled up so that the device finds its way into the Schlemm's canal. If the bevel is positioned to facilitate a "direct" insertion into the Schlemm's canal (parallel to iris root) this may result in the implant going downwards damaging the angular structures or even the ciliary body and the iris.

Occasionally if resistance is found and the implant does not progress smoothly during implantation, the device should not be released. Sometimes if the device is stuck, movement is transferred to the inserter, moving it in the opposite direction to the injection movement thus exposing the implant that should remain in the same position, as it is not being introduced further in the Schlemm's canal. It is very important to recognize this situation and retract the device into the inserter again. The first step is to check the insertion angle and if after a second attempt, the device is stuck in the same place a good option is to move to another area even if a new incision is needed. In any case, the implant should not be released until the surgeon is sure that it is correctly and completely implanted in the canal. Although the device can be pushed into the Schlemm's or pulled out with a manipulator or a blunt instrument, these maneuvers are only effective when correcting a minor positioning problem. If any of the windows of the implant are even partially seen in the anterior chamber, removal of the device should be considered. If trabecular damage is not significant, the surgeon can consider implanting a second one. Depending on the damaged area it may be necessary to target or find another implantation site (Fig. 2.2).

Adequate position of the implant should be checked after implantation. As some bleeding is very common sometimes it might be necessary to remove the viscoelastic and the blood. Although not always possible, it is recommended to check the whole implant from the distal end to inlet.

Tearing of the trabecular meshwork If the grip is not firm enough or there are movements during the insertion, the device may rupture the trabecular meshwork

Fig. 2.2 Incomplete/incorrect placement of Hydrus implant, with most of the implant in the anterior chamber

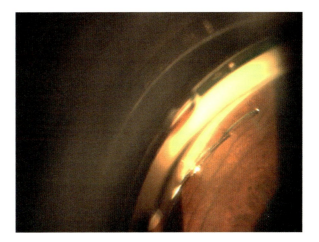

exposing the external wall of the Schlemm's canal. If there is not much bleeding a second implantation attempt can be performed.

Supraciliary/suprachoroidal implantation As in the case of the iStent, if the angle structures are not correctly identified there is an increased risk of damaging the ocular structures. The implantation of a device like this in the ciliary body is painful and involves a high risk of severe bleeding. It is important to recognize this situation as soon as the implant starts to dissect the ciliary body tissue and retract the device into the inserter. If the implant was completely released it should be removed using retina forceps. Depending on the ocular situation and the possible damage to the ciliary body and iris a new device could be implanted.

Iris or lens damage Rupture of the iris During the surgical procedure the surgeon should visualize the tip of the inserter and be careful to avoid touching the lens (in phakic eyes), cornea or the iris. Extra movements or surgical maneuvers increase the risk of damaging the ocular structures. If these maneuvers are needed for any reason, correct visualization is key to prevent further damage. If the device has to be removed, it is important to proceed slowly and control both ends of the device, also forceps should be used with care to avoid capturing the iris. If visualization of the device and/or angular structures is not good enough (blood or mixture of viscoelastic and blood), it can be improved by waiting for the bleeding to stop and then washing out the blood and viscoelastic.

Early Postoperative Complications
Hyphema Some bleeding is common and is not usually a problem. Pfeiffer et al. did not report any severe complications related to bleeding.

Malposition If for any reason, the position of the device could not be checked intraoperatively it should be as soon as possible. If the device is dislocated, or partially out of the Schlemm's canal it is probably better to remove it. Depending on the ocular conditions and IOP a new device can be implanted in the same surgery.

Late Postoperative Complications
There is little published evidence on the long-term complications; however, this device seems to be very safe.

Corneal Endothelial Cell damage If the surgery is uneventful and the device position correct, the possibility of significant endothelial damage is very low.

Peripheral Anterior Synechiae (PAS) and Inlet Obstruction Pfeiffer et al. reported that 18.8 % of patients may develop anterior synechiae after 2 years. These PAS were located at or near the inlet segment of the implant and consisted in focal iris tissue adhesion to the device or chamber angle usually of less than 1 clock hour. However, PAS did not have a negative impact on the success rate. In this series, no cases of complete blockage of the inlet by the iris were found.

2.2.3 Trabectome

The Trabectome (NeoMedix, Tustin, USA) is designed to electrosurgically ablate the trabecular meshwork and inner wall of Schlemm's canal. This enables aqueous to bypass the juxtacanalicular trabecular meshwork and inner wall of Schlemm's canal, which is thought to be the main site of resistance in open-angle glaucoma (Overby et al. 2009).

2.2.3.1 Safety and Efficacy
Results from the use of the Trabectome were first reported by Minckler et al. (2005). Company data for 4659 treatments show that it safely reduces the need for drops for several years and reduces IOP by 26 % (Mosaed 2014). A retrospective study suggested that Trabectome is less effective than trabeculectomy (Jea et al. 2012a). To date, there are no published randomized controlled trial data.

Rates of successful IOP control decline with time, particularly in the first year postoperatively (Ahuja ct al. 2013; Minckler et al. 2008; Mosaed 2014). Success rates reported in case series vary from 64 % to over 80 % at 12 months postoperatively, and from 62 % to more than 75 % at 24 months. Interpretation of results is hampered by the absence of clear criteria for the use of IOP-lowering medications in the postoperative period and by loss to follow-up of a significant proportion of patients.

Trabectome treatment may be more effective when combined with cataract surgery (Ahuja et al. 2013; Francis 2010; Jordan et al. 2013). Phacoemulsification itself has been shown to lower IOP (Chen et al. 2015; Mansberger et al. 2012), and the relative contributions of Trabectome and phacoemulsification are not yet defined by randomized trials.

Recently, it has been reported that Trabectome treatment may be effective in relatively narrow angles (Bussel et al. 2015a) and also in patients after failed trabeculectomy (Bussel et al. 2015b). Trabectome does not violate the integrity of the conjunctiva, and one cohort study suggests that the success of subsequent trabeculectomy is not compromised (Jea et al. 2012b).

In a single-center case series (Ahuja et al. 2013), the commonest complications were hyphema (46 %), microhyphema (27 %), and IOP spike (22 %). Other complications that have been reported include reduction in visual acuity >2 lines (0–5 %) (Ahuja et al. 2013; Minckler et al. 2008), delayed onset hyphema (5 %) (Ahuja et al. 2012), and aqueous misdirection (0.4 %) (Ahuja et al. 2013). In the manufacturer's case series (Mosaed 2014), hypotony (IOP < 5 mmHg) at day 1 occurred in 1 % but sustained hypotony at 1 month was rare (0.2 %). Secondary surgery was required in 7 % of cases.

2.2.3.2 Patient Selection and Procedure

Trabectome surgery may be performed under local anesthesia. The Trabectome probe consists of an irrigating-aspirating handpiece which is introduced into the anterior chamber through a 1.6 mm temporal incision in clear cornea. Under gonioscopic guidance, the end of the probe is advanced across the anterior chamber towards the nasal trabecular meshwork. The footplate of the probe is inserted through the trabecular meshwork into the lumen of the nasal part of Schlemm's canal. The footplate is then advanced along the lumen of Schlemm's canal while electrosurgical power is applied to ablate the inner wall of Schlemm's canal and the overlying trabecular meshwork.

Phacoemulsification can be performed after the Trabectome surgery through the same corneal incision, following enlargement, or via a separately placed incision. Some surgeons argue that phacoemulsification should be performed prior to Trabectome surgery, not afterwards. This way, the surgical view is less likely to be compromised by blood reflux following Trabectome surgery and the drainage angle may be more open and accessible. On the other hand, any reduction in corneal clarity at the end of phacoemulsification is likely to produce a poor gonioscopic view for Trabectome surgery.

Patients need to have surgically visible and accessible nasal drainage angles. To permit a gonioscopic view of the drainage angle, the patient must be able to rotate his or her head away from the surgeon. Inability to do this is a contraindication for surgery. Similarly, corneal opacities are a relative contraindication to surgery. Angles that appear to be relatively narrow on gonioscopy in the clinic may nonetheless be accessible surgically because the pressure of irrigation from the handpiece causes the lens-iris diaphragm to move posteriorly. However, angles that have peripheral anterior synechiae are unlikely to be amenable to treatment, because the iris tissue may not ablate easily and is liable to bleed heavily. The pupil is usually dilated if combined Trabectome-phacoemulsification is planned. Otherwise, preoperative application of pilocarpine eye drops may assist with opening the drainage angle. Through miosis, folds of iris are moved away from the ablation site and the crystalline lens is relatively protected from trauma. If, despite these precautions, iris is being aspirated into the handpiece, the surgeon should reduce the aspiration flow rate.

It is advisable to deflate the anterior chamber prior to introduction of the Trabectome probe. This allows blood to reflux into Schlemm's canal from the collector channels, thereby permitting easier identification of the canal, particularly in unpigmented angles. Although the blood may drain back into the collector channels following pressurization of the eye by the irrigating Trabectome probe, the operator will have had an opportunity to identify the location of the Schlemm's canal.

In order to minimize the risk of trauma to the crystalline lens, cornea or iris, the surgeon should hold the handpiece in such a way that the tip can be comfortably manipulated in the fingers of one hand. Electrosurgical power should never be activated when the tip of the probe is dry as this may cause damage to the handpiece.

Rotating the goniolens with one hand and the eye using the handpiece will enable a greater length of the nasal trabecular meshwork to be visualized. Thus, the potentially treatable area can be maximized.

Reflux of blood from the collector channels into the anterior chamber following removal of the irrigating handpiece from the eye is to be expected. Indeed, such reflux is regarded as a sign of correct ablation, and helps to identify the extent of ablation. The surgeon should quickly repressurize the eye to tamponade the reflux. Viscoelastic may be used as the tamponading agent if the next step is phacoemulsification. The viscoelastic is injected so as to displace blood, maintaining the red reflex for the capsulorhexis to be performed.

Following surgery, IOP-lowering drops should be continued. They may be cautiously withdrawn some weeks or months postoperatively if surgery has been performed as a drop-sparing procedure for patients who are allergic to or intolerant of one or more eye drops. Patients should be prescribed a course of topical steroids, antibiotics, and pilocarpine. The pilocarpine drops are intended to prevent the formation of peripheral anterior synechiae, which may occlude the opening in Schlemm's canal.

Blood is commonly noted in the angle or on the iris at day 1 postoperatively. However, it has usually cleared by week 1 (Minckler et al. 2005). Patients should be counseled preoperatively that their vision may be blurred in the first week owing to the reflux of blood into the anterior chamber.

2.2.3.3 Complications

Intraoperative Complications

Poor Visibility

Excellent visibility of the area to be treated is key to the success of the procedure. The surgeon must use adequately high microscope magnification when introducing the footplate into Schlemm's canal and when ablating tissue. Bubbles of air between the goniolens and the cornea are to be avoided through the use of sufficient coupling medium. However, care should be taken to avoid contaminating the top surface of the goniolens with the coupling medium, as this will reduce visibility. Equally, the manufacturer's instructions for setting up the equipment need to be followed meticulously to avoid introducing air into the anterior chamber via the handpiece during the procedure. Air bubbles in the anterior chamber will block the surgeon's view. As the handpiece's own aspiration function is insufficient to remove intracameral air, the handpiece needs to be removed in order for the air to be exchanged first with viscoelastic and then with balanced salt solution. Surgeons are advised to avoid using the Trabectome probe with viscoelastic in the anterior chamber as this may adversely affect heat dissipation.

Insertion of Footplate

To minimize any difficulty introducing the footplate into the lumen of Schlemm's canal, the surgeon should insert the footplate through the trabecular meshwork at a point that is not directly opposite the corneal incision. In this way, the tip of the footplate is directed obliquely (and not parallel to) the plane of the trabecular meshwork. It is also important to ensure that the tip of the footplate is not inadvertently bent or blunted by contact with hard surfaces. Particular care should be taken to avoid damaging the footplate during the removal of the plastic cap from the end of the handpiece.

Incomplete Ablation

Incomplete ablation occurs if the footplate of the probe is not introduced properly into the lumen of Schlemm's canal. Clean ablation of tissue is thought to be important to prevent resealing and closure of Schlemm's canal. Before starting ablation, the surgeon should verify correct placement of the footplate by gently tenting up the tissue with the probe. During ablation, the surgeon must ensure that sufficient electrosurgical power is applied. Application of insufficient power may result in tearing of the tissues and clogging of the tip with tissue. On the other hand, application of excessive power risks thermal damage to Schlemm's canal and the orifices of the collector channels. Visible charring of tissues is an indication for treatment power to be reduced. Following ablation, the deroofed Schlemm's canal should be visible as a shiny white gutter. It can be helpful to use the blunt heel of the footplate as a manipulator to verify that the canal has been successfully deroofed. Parts of the canal that have not been deroofed successfully may be retreated, with care to avoid thermal damage.

False Passage

False passage with damage to Schlemm's canal can be avoided by verifying correct placement of the footplate before starting ablation. Because the tissue to be ablated is quite thin, it should be easily tented up with the probe. Also, there should be minimal resistance to the advancement of the probe. Resistance may signify that the tip of the probe is misdirected and has engaged the outer wall of Schlemm's canal. The surgeon should reorientate the probe.

Bleeding

During ablation, the pressure of irrigation prevents blood reflux from the collector channels. Therefore, overt bleeding suggests that a vessel containing blood at arterial pressure has been damaged. This may be due to an unintentionally posterior ablation at the iris root, or due to unrecognized vascular tissue overlying the trabecular meshwork. Regardless of the cause of the bleeding, the surgeon needs to assess quickly whether blood is going to prevent proper visualization of the drainage angle. If so, the Trabectome procedure cannot be completed. The Trabectome probe should be withdrawn and the bleeding tamponaded immediately with viscoelastic injected into the anterior chamber. Once done, the surgeon may cautiously evaluate whether clotting has occurred by exchanging the viscoelastic for balanced salt solution. If so, there is the option to proceed with phacoemulsification (if this was planned). Otherwise, the eye should be closed and managed for hyphema.

Cyclodialysis Cleft

A cyclodialysis cleft may be created if ablation is performed too posteriorly, at the root of the iris. This may be heralded by bleeding, or by the appearance of the iris falling posteriorly. Unless there is bleeding, this complication may be managed conservatively, at least initially. A low intraocular pressure is to be expected at day 1 and in the first few weeks postoperatively. Indeed, an unexpectedly low intraocular pressure found postoperatively is reason to suspect that a cyclodialysis cleft has been created. Some surgeons withhold pilocarpine postoperatively to encourage the cleft to heal. Small clefts heal spontaneously. Large ones may require formal repair. Anterior segment imaging techniques such as optical coherence tomography may allow the size of clefts to be quantified.

Descemet's Membrane Detachment

Detachment of Descemet's membrane may occur if the ablation is performed too anteriorly or if the trabecular meshwork tissues are being torn rather than ablated. The measures to ensure correct placement of the ablation and to avoid tearing tissue have been outlined previously. If the detachment is small and confined to the peripheral cornea, it is unlikely that visually significant corneal edema will develop.

Trauma to Lens, Iris or Cornea

In order to minimize the risk of trauma to the crystalline lens, iris or cornea, the surgeon should hold the handpiece in such a way that the tip can be comfortably manipulated in the fingers of one hand. The probe needs to be passed across the anterior chamber with due care, ensuring that the handpiece irrigation is switched on continuously. The surgeon needs to be prepared to perform lens extraction should the capsule of the crystalline lens be inadvertently punctured during Trabectome surgery.

Early Postoperative Complications

Bleeding
The presence of a microhyphema or clotted blood in the angle or on the iris is to be expected immediately after surgery. Early postoperative hyphema is reported in 46 % of cases (Ahuja et al. 2013), but unless it is large should probably not be considered a complication of surgery.

IOP Spike
A spike in intraocular pressure of greater than 10 mmHg has been reported in 6–22 % of cases with a median onset of 34 days (Ahuja et al. 2013; Minckler et al. 2008). To avoid this, patients' usual IOP-lowering eye drops should not be withdrawn in the early postoperative period.

Hypotony
Early postoperative hypotony should cause the surgeon to suspect that a cyclodialysis cleft has been created. This may be verified gonioscopically or by use of anterior segment imaging such as optical coherence tomography. Some surgeons withhold pilocarpine postoperatively to encourage the cleft to heal. Small clefts heal spontaneously, whereas large ones may require formal repair.

Late Postoperative Complications

Bleeding
Spontaneous late bleeding, occurring more than 2 months postoperatively and sometimes recurrent, has been reported by different authors (Ahuja et al. 2012; Kassam et al. 2014). In one case series (Ahuja et al. 2012), bleeding occurred in 5 % (12 of 262 cases). All patients had noted a transient decrease in vision, mostly on waking. Only one case required secondary surgical intervention in the form of trabeculectomy for refractory high IOP. The remainder were managed conservatively with steroid eye drops, with resolution of the hyphema within 2 weeks. Laser coagulation of collector channel orifices has also been employed (Kassam et al. 2014). Some authors have advocated discontinuation of anticoagulants prior to surgery (Minckler et al. 2005). Bleeding during and after subsequent trabeculectomy has also been reported (Kassam et al. 2014; Knape and Smith 2010).

Failure of IOP Control
Secondary surgery is reported to be required in 7 % of cases (Mosaed 2014), with the commonest secondary procedures being trabeculectomy (4 %) and aqueous shunt insertion (2 %). Trabectome treatment does not violate the integrity of the conjunctiva, and one cohort study suggested that failed Trabectome surgery does not compromise the likelihood of success of subsequent trabeculectomy (Jea et al. 2012b).

Practical Tip: Trans-trabecular Meshwork Surgeries

- Anterior vitrectomy should be performed if there is any chance of vitreous loss into the AC from previous surgery. Positioning of head of patient and tilting the microscope are essential for good visualization.
- Blood reflux into the anterior chamber is NOT a complication, it simply signals a direct communication between the anterior chamber and collectors had been established.
- Membrane formation covering the inlets of iStent & Hydrus as well as exposed collector channels after Trabectome surgery may benefit from YAG laser disruption.

2.3 Suprachoroidal Implants

2.3.1 CyPass

2.3.1.1 Safety and Efficacy

The CyPass Micro-Stent (Alcon Inc., Fort Worth, Texas, USA) is implanted into the supraciliary space to provide a permanent drainage conduit for aqueous along the suprachoroidal pathway (Saheb et al. 2014) (Fig. 2.3).

In a multicenter single-arm interventional study, patients with open-angle glaucoma and uncontrolled medicated intraocular pressure >21 mmHg at baseline were enrolled to receive CyPass Micro-Stent implantation alone (Garcia-Feijoo et al. 2015). Of 65 eyes treated, results for 55 were available at 12 months owing to loss to follow-up and early termination. Mean IOP decreased by 35 % from 24.5 mmHg at baseline to 16.4 mmHg at 12 months. Mean number of medications also reduced from 2.2 at baseline to 1.4 at 12 months. Of 64 eyes that were originally indicated for conventional glaucoma surgery, 83 % did not require secondary surgery at 1 year. The commonest adverse events were cataract progression (12 %), IOP increases > 30 mmHg beyond 1 month (11 %), and transient hyphema (6 %).

In a separate study examining the implantation of CyPass combined with phacoemulsification (Hoeh et al. 2016), patients who had open-angle glaucoma with IOP of 21 mmHg or higher despite topical medication or prior surgical glaucoma treatment (cohort 1) were analyzed separately from those who had IOP <21 mmHg with medical treatment (cohort 2). For cohort 1, there was a reduction in mean IOP from 25.9 mmHg at baseline to 16.2 mmHg at 3 months. The IOP-lowering effect was sustained at 12 months. The mean number of glaucoma medications was also reduced from 2.1 at baseline to 1.1 at 12 months. Although no IOP-lowering effect was found for cohort 2, there was a 75 % reduction in mean number of medications prescribed at 12 months, with 65 % of the patients still in the study at 12 months being medication-free. Interpretation of these results is hampered by the lack of

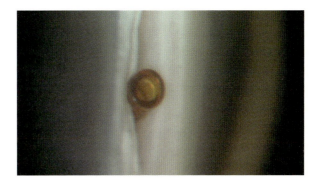

Fig. 2.3 A CyPass in its correct position in the anterior chamber

prespecified criteria for the management of IOP-lowering medications, the absence of a control group receiving phacoemulsification alone and by loss to follow-up. 25 of 65 patients in cohort 1 and 31 of 102 patients in cohort 2 were not followed up at 12 months. In terms of adverse events, 14 % of treated eyes had transient hypotony (IOP < 6 mmHg) which resolved by 1 month without visual sequelae. Elevated IOP > 30 mmHg and more than 9 mmHg above baseline occurred in 3 % of patients overall. Other complications included partial or complete obstruction of the implant (5 %) and endothelial touch (1 %). Secondary surgery, including stent repositioning, explantation or penetrating glaucoma surgery was required in 6 %.

2.3.1.2   Patient Selection and Procedure

The CyPass is a 6.35 mm long fenestrated stent made of polyimide. The device has three retention rings in its proximal end. These in combination with the fenestrations ensure the stability of the implant in the supraciliary space. It is threaded on a curved guide wire to facilitate its implantation into the suprachoroidal space following the scleral curvature. The guide wire tip is blunt to minimize the risk of tissue damage. The first step in the surgical procedure is to thread the CyPass on the retractable guide wire of the inserter.

The procedure can be performed under topical anesthesia and the setup (positioning of the patient's head and microscope and use of goniolens) is the same as in the angular surgeries described above. The implantation is usually performed using a 1.5 mm clear corneal incision opposite to the place where implantation is planned. Smaller incisions can be considered, as no lateral movements are required. When performed in combination with phacoemulsification the same incision can be used. The injection of acetylcholine is recommended then filling the anterior chamber with a viscoelastic agent to open the angle and improve access to the iris insertion. The CyPass inserter is then introduced in the anterior chamber and directed to the iris root aiming at the iris insertion just below the ciliary band. The suprachoidal space is virtual and the small rupture of the iris root and the creation of the dissection plane between the ciliary body and the sclera is easily done with the blunt tip of the guide wire. If resistance is found it is most likely that the angle of insertion is too flat (too parallel to the iris plane) so the tip hits the sclera. If this occurs the insertion angle should be increased to facilitate the access to the suprachoroidal space. If the insertion angle is correct, very little resistance to the inserter advance is to be expected. The CyPass should be introduced until only two retention rings are seen, then the guide wire is retracted leaving the device in place and the inserter can be withdrawn. Some bleeding is common and usually does not interfere with the surgical procedure. Surgery is completed with the removal of the viscoelastic agent and the blood. At the end of surgery it is recommended to check the position of the CyPass: Ideally just two of the retention rings should be visualized in the anterior chamber.

The advantage of a procedure that uses the suprachoroidal drainage is that the efficacy is not limited by the condition of the posttrabecular outflow system. But an accessible and sufficiently open-angle is required to prevent the CyPass touching the cornea or come too close to the corneal endothelium. The indications of this procedure are potentially wider than trabecular/Schlemm's Canal surgeries and include secondary open-angle glaucoma. Garcia-Feijoo et al. reported that after 1 year 25 % of the patients achieved an IOP < 13 mm Hg. If this data is confirmed, and given the safety profile of the procedure, CyPass implantation could be considered in more advanced glaucoma cases or after filtration surgery failures. However, the success rate of these possible indications is still to be established.

2.3.1.3   Complications

Intraoperative Complications
In the majority of cases, intraoperative complications arise owing to an inappropriate surgical procedure. So it is most important that an adequate visualization of the angle is obtained and the implant is inserted at the correct angle.

Inadequate position of the CyPass   If the CyPass is too deep or too superficial, it may cause problems. The recommendation is to check the position of the implant once surgery is complete. If it is too deep the anterior opening could be blocked by the iris/ciliary body tissue, the created opening may close leading to a surgical failure. On the other hand if the implant is too anterior it may come into contact with the cornea damaging the corneal endothelium. If malposition is evidenced during surgery the device can be repositioned using retinal forceps.

Bleeding   This is one of the most frequent complications arising during surgery. Some slight bleeding can be expected given that a small perforation has to be made in the iris. In order to prevent excessive bleeding the implant should be inserted while avoiding lateral movements. Also if patent iris vessels are seen close to the angle or running parallel to the iris root, this area should be avoided.

Cyclodialysis. Disinsertion of the Iris   For the CyPass insertion no lateral movements are required and should be avoided. Lateral movements during insertion not only increase the chances of significant bleeding but also could cause sectorial disinsertion of the iris. In this case a wide area of direct communication between the anterior chamber and the suprachoroid space will be created thus increasing the chances of hypotony or choroidal detachment.

Ciliary Body Damage Although this is theoretically possible, the inserter curvature has been designed to follow the scleral curvature and also the point of the guide wire is blunt making it very difficult to penetrate the ciliary body tissue. In the published papers no relevant damage to the ciliary body has been reported.

Early Postoperative Complications
Early complications are mostly related to the surgical procedure. After uneventful surgery complications are infrequent but can include hyphema, iris damage or disinsertion, and endothelial damage. Choroid effusion or detachment is a potential risk in any anti-glaucoma surgical technique and more so in surgery that involves the suprachoroid space as an evacuation route for the aqueous humor.

Hyphema As mentioned above in a multicenter single-arm interventional study, around 7 % of the patients had a transient hyphema that resolved in the first month. Excessive manipulation of the iris root/supraciliary space and specifically lateral movements could increase the risk of severe bleeding.

Suprachoidal Hemorrahage This is a risk in any anti-glaucoma surgery and it could be speculated that might be more likely in suprachoridal surgeries. However, in the published series this complication has not reported. So it seems that the risk of having this complication is very low.

IOP spikes In the mentioned follow-up study by Garcia-Feijoo et al., the authors defined as transient IOP elevation after surgery an IOP >30 mm Hg during a study visit but that resolved either on its own or with reintroduction of glaucoma medications on a subsequent visit. These transient spikes were observed in 10.8 % of the cases. It can be hypothesized that the spikes could be related to the scar tissue covering the device. Most of the cases resolved with glaucoma medication.

Hypotony This is a possible complication of any suprachoidal surgery, although no cases of hypotony have been reported.

Late Postoperative Complications
We lack published evidence on long-term complications, as the follow-up of the published series is short.

CyPass Displacement The combination of the fenestrations, the retention rings and the scarring response around the device result in the stabilization of the device in position. However, migration of the device is theoretically possible. An anterior migration could result in a device touching the cornea or coming too close to the endothelium. On the other hand, posterior migration could introduce the CyPass deep in the suprachoroidal space facilitating the obstruction of the CyPass by the iris. Anterior migration could be more likely and intrasurgical incorrect positioning and/or excessive scarring/scarring response around the device might play a role in the displacement of the CyPass.

Corneal Endothelial Damage An anterior position of the anterior tip of the CyPass can result in endothelial damage. There are no data on the long-term repercussion on the corneal endothelium of well positioned devices.

IOP Spikes As mentioned before the failure of the surgery can be associated with an IOP spike. Garcia-Feijoo et al. reported that 16.9 % of the patients needed additional surgery to control the IOP (second CyPass or trabeculectomy).

Obstruction of the CyPass/Synechia The iris can partially or totally obstruct the anterior opening of the device. In these cases Nd-YAG laser can be used to clear the synechia. This complication is more likely if the device was inserted too deep. If this is the case surgical repositioning of the CyPass could be necessary.

Practical Tip: Suprachoroidal Implants
Positioning of head of patient and tilting the microscope are essential for good visualization.
    Membrane formation covering the inlets of Suprachoroidal implant may occur.

2.4   Subconjunctival Implants

2.4.1   XEN Gel Implant

2.4.1.1   Safety and Efficacy
The Xen Gel Implant (Allergan, Dublin, Ireland) is a 6 mm long porcine collagen implant cross-linked to prevent degradation. It is designed to be injected *ab interno* from the anterior chamber to drain into the subconjunctival or subtenon's space. No safety or efficacy data have yet been published in peer-reviewed journals. Two industry-sponsored studies are ongoing (Clinicaltrials.gov NCT02036541 and NCT02006693), but neither is a randomized controlled trial.

A recent conference poster (Rekas et al. 2014) reported outcomes from 107 subjects. The mean preoperative, best medicated IOP was 21.8 mmHg. Mean postoperative IOPs were 15.9 at 12 months, 15.1 at 18 months, and 14.2 at 24 months. Anti-glaucomatous medications were reduced from the preoperative median of 2.8 (patients not washed out presurgery) by 64 % at 12 and 18 months, and by 57 % at 24 months. 6 % had secondary glaucoma surgery by 24 months, but no major adverse events were reported.

In another conference report (Reitsamer 2014), 74 patients had preoperative Mitomycin C (MMC) injection followed by XEN implantation, with or without concomitant cataract surgery. The mean preoperative, best medicated IOP was 22.3 mmHg (patients not washed out presurgery). Mean postoperative IOPs were 15.5 mmHg at 3 months, 14.9 mmHg at 6 months, and 14.7 mmHg at 9 months, though not all patients had reached 9 months of follow-up. Mean number of preoperative anti-glaucoma medications was 3.2, and was reduced to 0.5 at 3 months, 1.0 at 6 months, and 0.8 at 9 months. No secondary glaucoma surgery or major adverse events were reported by 9 months.

2.4.1.2 Patient Selection and Procedure

The Xen Gel Implant, because of its apparently greater pressure-lowering efficacy, is an alternative to trabeculectomy as a standalone procedure in a proportion of patients. As it is seems less likely to achieve low long-term IOP levels than trabeculectomy, but does have greater IOP-lowering efficacy than TM procedures, the Xen seems most appropriate for those with significant IOP elevation who do not have very advanced glaucoma and hence do not need very low target IOPs.

On the other hand, when used in combination with phaco, the converse argument might be that the Xen, because of its greater potential pressure-lowering efficacy, might be more appropriate than TM procedures.

Xen implantation differs from the trabecular meshwork procedures in that, by consensus view, Mitomycin C (MMC) injection is required just before implantation to reduce the subconjunctival healing response. A common contemporary technique is to inject 0.1 ml of 0.2 mg/ml MMC to the superior subconjunctival space away from the limbus, just before implantation. The MMC bleb can then be massaged gently to the superonasal subconjunctival space. Injecting away from the limbus and superiorly, rather than superonasally is intended to avoid creating a very avascular bleb close to the limbus in the inter-palpebral conjunctiva.

The superonasal conjunctiva is then dried with a sponge and ink marks made 3 mm from the limbus to indicate the target zone for the implantation.

A corneal paracentesis is made inferotemporally 1 mm into clear cornea from the limbus. A second paracentesis is made superotemporally for a second instrument such as a Vera Hook or iris repositor. If an iris repositor is to be used as the second instrument, a helpful technique is to make a further paracentesis diagonally opposite to allow the iris repositor to transfix the globe. There are a few advantages to this as follows:

- While the Vera hook can be used to plug the side port tightly, this is not the case with the iris repositor or other types of second instrument that are loose and can move around. In general, while the surgeon is concentrating on the superior conjunctival area when injecting the Xen, a second instrument such as an iris repositor that is mobile will not provide stable fixation, and worse still maybe touch and traumatize intraocular structures such as lens and iris.

- Use of the iris repositor to transfix the globe facilitates rotation of the globe and implantation closer to the superior limbus and less nasal, reducing the likelihood of dysesthesia from a bleb below the upper lid.
- Use of the iris repositor in the above manner, protects the lens in phakic eyes from trauma from the injector if the patient moves suddenly during implantation.

After making the initial incisions, the anterior chamber is inflated using a visco-elastic such as Healon GV.

The injector is then briefly checked by advancing the Xen slightly to ensure the device is correctly loaded and then wet with a small amount of balanced salt solution. The Xen is then gently repositioned back to its original position and the injector introduced into the anterior chamber. A 20 gauge MVR blade incision just fits the Xen injector snugly so it may be necessary to wiggle from side to side to get the shoulder of the injector past the internal opening into the anterior chamber.

The injector is directed into the angle in a line aiming to traverse the angle and sclera in a line that would result in it exiting sclera just at the 3 mm mark from the limbus.

If a goniolens is to be used, it should be placed on the cornea at this juncture. It is impossible to perform gonioscopy and inject at the same time because of the need for counter-traction with a second instrument. The goniolens can be used to position the injector at the correct position in the angle if the position can be maintained while the lens is removed and the second instrument inserted. An indirect goniolens such as the Ahmed 1.5× Surgical Goniolens (Ocular Instruments, Bellevue, Washington, USA) is most suitable for this.

After checking the position of the injector tip in the angle on gonioscopy, the goniolens is removed and the second instrument positioned via the side port. Gentle pressure is then applied to advance the injector through sclera, taking care not to advance the slider or inject. As the injector advances, it is important to attempt to direct it so that it emerges from sclera at the level of the 3 mm marks. If it emerges anterior to the marks, the result will be a more corneal injection. Behind the marks will result in an implantation closer to iris, potentially traversing suprachoroidal space before traversing sclera. If the implant is too close to iris, there is a greater chance of iris occlusion. If the injector appears to be exiting sclera too far forward or back, then it is a simple matter to withdraw into the anterior chamber, reposition and re-advance.

Once the injector tip has exited sclera in the correct plane and is visible subconjunctivally, it is worth advancing slightly further to ensure that the injected implant does not get stuck in episclera. The injector is then rotated through 90 degrees either clockwise or anticlockwise. At this point the slider on the injector is slowly advanced to inject the implant. It is important to maintain forward pressure with the injector at this point to prevent the injector sliding back into the anterior chamber prematurely. Once the slider has moved the full length of its travel, the needle tip will have retracted and the implant should be visible in the subconjunctival or subtenon's space.

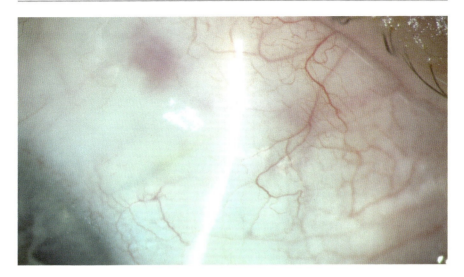

Fig. 2.4 A diffuse subconjunctival bleb surrounding a Xen implant

At this point the viscoelastic should be removed from the anterior chamber using either a manual or automatic irrigation system. One should then be able to see a bleb developing over the device in the subconjunctival space.

If no bleb is visible, one should firstly look at the device. If the device is curled up in a *pigtail* appearance, it may be embedded in Tenon's capsule and the external aperture obstructed by Tenon's. This can be remedied by taking a pair of tying forceps and gently stroking the implant to straighten it. Often a bleb will start to appear at that point. If the tube is deemed to be too long, it can be fed back towards the anterior chamber using the forceps and vice versa if it is too short (Fig. 2.4).

If no bleb is still visible it is worth performing gonioscopy again to ensure that the anterior chamber positioning is correct and the tube is patent at its internal ostium.

2.4.1.3 Complications

Intraoperative Complications
Intraoperative complications with Xen relate either to difficulty with implant positioning or hyphema. In phakic eyes, the potential for lens touch exists, e.g., if the patient moves during surgery. Management of hyphema and avoidance of lens touch are as for the procedures previously described.

Early Postoperative Complications
Apart from hyphema and rarely infection, the risks in the early postoperative period are low pressure and high pressure. Low IOP is not uncommon, especially in younger patients. Significant anterior chamber shallowing is relatively uncommon but occasionally requires topical atropine or serial injections of viscoelastic in out-patients. In the author's experience (KB), hypotony does not last more than 2 weeks in the most extreme case.

High IOP during the first few days might be indicative of retained viscoelastic, but more likely occurs from obstruction of the Xen, either externally by Tenon's, or occasionally internally, by iris.

Late Postoperative Complications
As the Xen has only been available for just over 2 years, long-term experience is almost non-existent. Dysesthesia, blebitis, and endophthalmitis are a possibility though they seem to be rare. One of the authors (KB) has experienced two cases of implant exposure in around 120 cases, both necessitating implant removal. Other than that, the longer term risk is failure of IOP control, but much greater experience will be required to quantify this accurately.

2.4.2 MicroShunt

The MicroShunt (Innfocus, Miami, Florida, USA) is an 8.5 mm flexible tube of 70 μm lumen diameter made from a polyolefin triblock polymer (poly(Styrene-block-IsoButylene-block-Styrene)) that is designed to drain from the anterior chamber to the subtenons space behind the limbus. In that respect, the mode of action is similar to the Xen. However, the MicroShunt differs from the Xen and any other MIGS-type procedure in that it is implanted via an *ab externo* approach. Although some would regard this as a disadvantage, the mode of implantation does benefit from minimal anterior chamber intervention, making it an attractive proposition in stand-alone cases that are not undergoing concomitant cataract surgery.

2.4.2.1 Safety and Efficacy
At the time of writing, there are no published high-quality trials of MicroShunt safety and efficacy in peer-reviewed journals but a US and European randomized surgical trial is underway with the stated objective to obtain FDA approval as an alternative to trabeculectomy.

2.4.2.2 Patient Selection and Procedure
Implantation of the MicroShunt is believed to be indicated in patients who would otherwise be suitable for trabeculectomy. The absence of published high-quality evidence at present makes this difficult to verify.

The implantation procedure involves making a superior limbal conjunctival incision at the 12 o'clock position, similar to that for trabeculectomy. A subtenon's dissection is made in order to open up the subtenon's space for MMC application. Light cautery is applied to the episclera to achieve hemostasis in order to ensure that contact with blood does not blunt the effect of the MMC. MMC is applied in a similar fashion to a trabeculectomy procedure on a number of sponges over a wide area. The MMC is then irrigated away using 20 ml of BSS.

A point 3 mm behind the limbus is then marked with ink. A scleral tunnel is then created with a 1 mm diameter slit knife that is advanced 2 mm to a predefined mark. The slit knife is then withdrawn and a 25 gauge (orange) hypodermic needle gently

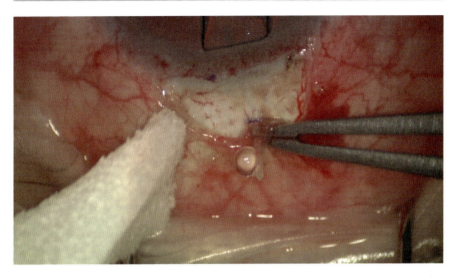

Fig. 2.5 Demonstration of aqueous flow through a Microshunt implant before conjunctival closure

inserted into the tunnel and advanced to its apex. The needle is then angled in order to advance it into the anterior chamber parallel to the plane of the iris and subsequently withdrawn.

The implant is washed with BSS in order to eliminate static electricity, gently grasped with tying forceps just in front of the fin and advanced into the anterior chamber via the tunnel. The Tunnel is designed in a manner to allow the fin to sit snugly intrasclerally. At this point, the tube portion should be visible in the anterior chamber, away from iris and cornea and the implant should be immobile in the tunnel without sutures.

It is important to ensure that the tube is draining aqueous before closure. This can be achieved by observing aqueous egress at the external aperture of the tube using a small sponge or fluorescein. If no flow is observed initially, it can usually be initiated by pressing on the eye gently at the limbus. If repeated firm pressure is insufficient to initiate flow, a wide bore, thin-walled 23 gauge cannula has been sourced by the manufacturer of the implant that can be placed over the length of the tube and used to flush it (Fig. 2.5).

After confirming that the implant is draining, the Tenon's and conjunctiva are closed. It is important before reapposing the conjunctiva at the limbus to ensure that Tenon's is lifted up over the implant and also brought towards the limbus. This is to ensure that the implant does not become caught in Tenon's or bent forward when conjunctiva and Tenon's are reapposed.

It is often helpful, where feasible, to suture conjunctiva and Tenon's separately. Firstly, one can ensure that Tenon's does not slip back around the implant. Secondly, this avoids drawing Tenon's right up to the limbus, which occasionally, if tight, can predispose to ptosis.

2.4.2.3   Complications

Intraoperative Complications
There are relatively few challenges with MicroShunt insertion. These include bleeding on needle insertion that might result in a postoperative hyphema, malpositioning of the shunt either in iris or cornea, which is simply remedied by removal and creation of a separate tunnel, and failure to observe flow the through the tube.

Early Postoperative Complications
Possibly early postoperative complications include hyphema, hypotony, or obstruction of the tube. To date these are all relatively uncommon. Hypotony is likely to be an issue in some patients as the internal diameter of the device at 70 μm does not provide sufficient resistance in a device 8.5 mm long to maintain intraocular pressure without some additional resistance from conjunctiva and Tenon's. The reported hypotony rate from company information is <10 % and all have been stated to resolve spontaneously within 1 week. The choroidal effusion rate has been reported to be 5 %.

Late Postoperative Complications
At the time of writing, there are no long-term reports upon which to assess safety or efficacy.

Practical Tip
- Start 2 mm from the limbus with a smooth single entry initially in the plane of the sclera then angling forward parallel with the iris plane once half of the bevel is in the sclera.
- Ensure a single movement without retraction and advancement (as this can create a false pocket).
- Enlarge the track slightly on exit to aid with initiating the tube entry.
- Check for watertight fit with 2 % fluorescein, suture adjacent to the tube if leaking.
- Persistent leaks may be stopped by plugging with Tenon's tissue.
- Ensure flow through the tube at the end of the surgeries. In the case of Xen, bleb formation is critical at the end of surgery.
- Bleb encapsulation can occur, and needling with 5-fluorouracil should be considered postoperatively.

References

Ahuja Y, Malihi M, Sit AJ. Delayed-onset symptomatic hyphema after ab interno trabeculotomy surgery. Am J Ophthalmol. 2012;154:476–80.e2.

Ahuja Y, Ma Khin Pyi S, Malihi M, et al. Clinical results of ab interno trabeculotomy using the trabectome for open-angle glaucoma: the Mayo Clinic series in Rochester, Minnesota. Am J Ophthalmol. 2013;156:927–935.e2.

Arriola-Villalobos P, Martínez-de-la-Casa JM, Díaz-Valle D, et al. Combined iStent trabecular micro-bypass stent implantation and phacoemulsification for coexistent open-angle glaucoma and cataract: a long-term study. Br J Ophthalmol. 2012;96(5):645–9.

Arriola-Villalobos P, Martínez-de-la-Casa JM, Díaz-Valle D, et al. Mid-term evaluation of the new Glaukos iStent with phacoemulsification in coexistent open-angle glaucoma or ocular hypertension and cataract. Br J Ophthalmol. 2013;97(10):1250–5.

Bussel II, Kaplowitz K, Schuman JS, et al. Outcomes of ab interno trabeculectomy with the trabectome by degree of angle opening. Br J Ophthalmol. 2015a;99:914–9.

Bussel II, Kaplowitz K, Schuman JS, et al. Outcomes of ab interno trabeculectomy with the trabectome after failed trabeculectomy. Br J Ophthalmol. 2015b;99:258–62.

Chen PP, Lin SC, Junk AK, et al. The effect of phacoemulsification on intraocular pressure in glaucoma patients: a report by the American Academy of Ophthalmology. Ophthalmology. 2015;22:1294–307.

Craven ER, Katz LJ, Wells JM, et al. Cataract surgery with trabecular micro-bypass stent implantation in patients with mild-to-moderate open-angle glaucoma and cataract: two-year follow-up. J Cataract Refract Surg. 2012;38:1339–45.

Fea AM. Phacoemulsification versus phacoemulsification with micro-bypass stent implantation in primary open-angle glaucoma: randomized double-masked clinical trial. J Cataract Refract Surg. 2010;36:407–12.

Fea AM, Belda JI, Rekas M, et al. Prospective unmasked randomized evaluation of the iStent inject ((R)) versus two ocular hypotensive agents in patients with primary open-angle glaucoma. Clin Ophthalmol. 2014;8:875–82.

Fernández-Barrientos Y, García-Feijoó J, Martínez-de-la-Casa JM, et al. Fluorophotometric study of the effect of the glaukos trabecular microbypass stent on aqueous humor dynamics. Invest Ophthalmol Vis Sci. 2010;51:3327–32.

Francis BA. Trabectome combined with phacoemulsification versus phacoemulsification alone: a prospective, non-randomized controlled surgical trial. Clin Surg Ophthalmol. 2010; 28:1–7.

Garcia-Feijoo J, Rau M, Grisanti S, et al. Supraciliary micro-stent implantation for open-angle glaucoma failing topical therapy: 1-year results of a multicenter study. Am J Ophthalmol. 2015;159:1075–1081.e1.

Hoeh H, Vold SD, Ahmed IK, et al. Initial clinical experience with the CyPass micro-stent: safety and surgical outcomes of a novel supraciliary microstent. J Glaucoma. 2016;25:106-12.

Jea SY, Francis BA, Vakili G, et al. Ab interno trabeculectomy versus trabeculectomy for open-angle glaucoma. Ophthalmology. 2012a;119:36–42.

Jea SY, Mosaed S, Vold SD, et al. Effect of a failed trabectome on subsequent trabeculectomy. J Glaucoma. 2012b;21:71–5.

Jordan JF, Wecker T, Van Oterendorp C, et al. Trabectome surgery for primary and secondary open angle glaucomas. Graefes Arch Clin Exp Ophthalmol. 2013;251:2753–60.

Kassam F, Stechschulte AC, Stiles MC, et al. Delayed spontaneous hyphemas after Ab interno trabeculectomy surgery for glaucoma. J Glaucoma. 2014;23:660–1.

Knape RM, Smith MF. Anterior chamber blood reflux during trabeculectomy in an eye with previous trabectome surgery. J Glaucoma. 2010;19:499–500.

Mansberger SL, Gordon MO, Jampel H, et al. Reduction in intraocular pressure after cataract extraction: the Ocular Hypertension Treatment Study. Ophthalmology. 2012;119:1826–31.

Minckler DS, Baerveldt G, Alfaro MR, et al. Clinical results with the Trabectome for treatment of open-angle glaucoma. Ophthalmology. 2005;112:962–7.

Minckler D, Mosaed S, Dustin L, et al. Trabectome (trabeculectomy-internal approach): additional experience and extended follow-up. Trans Am Ophthalmol Soc. 2008;106:149–59; discussion 159–60.

Morales-Fernandez L, Martinez-De-La-Casa JM, Garcia-Feijoo J, et al. Glaukos trabecular stent used to treat steroid-induced glaucoma. Eur J Ophthalmol. 2012;22(4):670–3.

Mosaed S. The first decade of global trabectome outcomes. Clin Surg Ophthalmol. 2014;32:21–9.

Overby DR, Stamer WD, Johnson M. The changing paradigm of outflow resistance generation: towards synergistic models of the JCT and inner wall endothelium. Exp Eye Res. 2009;88:656–70.

Pfeiffer N, Garcia-Feijoo J, Martinez-De-La-Casa JM, et al. A randomized trial of a Schlemm's canal microstent with phacoemulsification for reducing intraocular pressure in open-angle glaucoma. Ophthalmology. 2015;122:1283–93.

Reitsamer H. Early results of a minimally-invasive, ab-interno gelatin stent in combination with a preoperative Mitomycin C injection for the treatment of glaucoma. London: XXXII Congress of the ESCRS; 2014.

Rekas M, Lewczuk K, Jablonska J, et al. Two year follow-up data with a soft and permanent, minimally-invasive ab-interno subconjunctival implant in open-angle glaucoma subjects. London: XXXII Congress of the ESCRS; 2014.

Saheb H, Ianchulev T, Ahmed I. Optical coherence tomography of the suprachoroid after CyPass Micro-Stent implantation for the treatment of open-angle glaucoma. Br J Ophthalmol. 2014;98:19–23.

Samuelson TW, Katz LJ, Wells JM, et al. Randomized evaluation of the trabecular micro-bypass stent with phacoemulsification in patients with glaucoma and cataract. Ophthalmology. 2011;118:459–67.

Voskanyan L, Garcia-Feijoo J, Belda JI, et al. Prospective, unmasked evaluation of the iStent(R) inject system for open-angle glaucoma: synergy trial. Adv Ther. 2014;31:189–201.

Nonpenetrating Glaucoma Surgery (Deep Sclerectomy, Viscocanaloplasty, and Canaloplasty)

3

Jason Cheng, Kuang Hu, and Nitin Anand

3.1 Introduction

The aim of all nonpenetrating glaucoma surgery (NPGS) procedures is the creation of a filtration membrane, the trabeculo-Descemet's membrane (TDM). Aqueous filters into a subscleral space created by excising a deep scleral flap. The final route for aqueous outflow differs between the two NPGS procedures. It is thought to be the subconjunctival space and possibly the suprachoroidal space with deep sclerectomy (DS) and enhanced flow through the Schlemm's canal in viscocanaloplasty (VCT) and its variant, canaloplasty.

The earliest descriptions of DS are in the Russian literature. A form of NPGS, sinusotomy, was described by Krasnov (1968), who excised a scleral lamella directly over Schlemm's canal to expose its lumen. Krasnov noted that care was required to avoid damage to the inner wall of Schlemm's canal, which would convert the operation to a fistulizing procedure. He also stated that the anterior chamber should not empty during the course of surgery, thereby preventing serious complications. Zimmerman and Kooner and published a comparative trial comparing ab-externo trabeculectomy with trabeculectomy about 30 years ago (Zimmerman et al. 1984). Andre Mermoud popularized the current DS procedure in the 1990s. VCT (Stegmann et al. 1999) and canaloplasty were both originally described by Robert Stegmann (Stegmann 1995).

J. Cheng
KhooTeck Puat Hospital, Yishun, Singapore
e-mail: jdcheng@gmail.com

K. Hu
Moorfields Eye Hospital NHS Foundation Trust, London, UK

N. Anand (✉)
Cheltenham General and Gloucester Royal Hospitals, Gloucester, UK
e-mail: anand1604@gmail.com

F. Carbonaro, K. Sheng Lim (eds.), *Managing Complications in Glaucoma Surgery*,
DOI 10.1007/978-3-319-49416-6_3, © Springer International Publishing AG 2017

3.2   Procedure for NPGS

Deep sclerectomy (DS) is the prototype NPGS procedure. It is important to empha-
size that success of both VCT and canaloplasty is also dependent on the creation of
adequate filtration through the TDM. The surgeon has to be familiar with the anatomy of the limbus (Fig. 3.1). The most important landmark is the transition zone.
The SC canal is at the posterior edge of this gray zone. A fornix-based conjunctival
flap is dissected with posterior dissection of MMC is used. The superficial scleral
flap may be rectangular or trapezoid in shape, approximately one-third scleral thickness and 5 mm at the limbus. The flap dissection should start at least 3 mm behind
the posterior edge of the anatomical limbus and is continued 1–2 mm into clear
cornea (Fig. 3.2a). MMC is applied posteriorly and may be applied either before or
after outer sclera flap dissection. Concentrations of 0.2 mg/ml for 1–3 min are adequate for most situations (Fig. 3.2b). Subconjunctival bevacuzimab 0.5 mg at the
end of the procedure may be used in low-risk cases (Anand and Bong 2015). Cautery
should be used sparingly. Blood in the surgical field can be absorbed by PVA sponge
fragments.

The inner or deep scleral flap dissection is critical and must be done under high
magnification (×14). The edges are 1 mm inside and can be gradually deepened until
the choroid is visible at the posterior edge and the Schlemm's canal was incised at
the lateral edges (Fig. 3.2c). The dissection is done at 95 % thickness of the remaining sclera and the choroid should be visible though the sclera. The scleral fibers
become circumferentially oriented when the scleral spur is reached (Fig. 3.2d). The
lateral edges are then extended into the cornea (Fig. 3.2e, f). Dissection centrally
should be done with a PVA or cellulose spears. Sharp instruments should be avoided
at this stage. The deep flap is then dissected in the plane of the scleral spur, de-
roofing the Schlemm's canal and continued about 1 mm into clear cornea and
excised (Fig. 3.2h). JXT is then peeled with a blunt-tipped capsulorrhexis forceps to
ensure percolation of aqueous through the TDM (Fig. 3.2i). A spacer device may be
placed in the scleral bed and the superficial scleral flap is loosely sutured back with
1-2 10/0 nylon sutures. The conjunctiva was sutured onto the limbus with two 10/0
nylon radial interrupted sutures.

In VCT, high molecular weight hyaluronic acid (Healon GV®) is injected via a
small-caliber cannula into the SC (Fig. 3.3). The aim is to dilate the SC and perhaps create microperforations in the inner wall (Tamm et al. 2004). Canaloplasty
involves passing a microcatheter into the ostium of Schlemm's canal. The microcatheter incorporates an illuminated tip that can be observed transsclerally during
catheterization of the canal and a lumen through which viscoelastic was delivered
to dilate the canal. Once exposed at the opposite ostium, 10-0 prolene suture
(Ethicon Inc.) is tied to the distal tip of the microcatheter. The microcatheter was
then retracted, injecting Healon GV™. The catheter is removed and the suture is
tied tight exerting tension on the SC. The superficial flap is closure is watertight,
with 5-6 interrupted 10-0 prolene sutures in both VCT and canaloplasty. The aim
of the tight closure is to avoid subconjunctival flow of aqueous and direct flow into
the SC (Fig. 3.4).

Fig. 3.1 Anatomy of the limbus. *Top:* arrow with dashed line shows the anterior edge of the surgical limbus, the attachment of the conjunctiva to cornea. The *solid arrow* shows the posterior edge of the transition (*gray*) zone, the usual location of Schlemm's canal. *Middle*: conjunctival dissection reveals a wide transition zone. *Arrows* indicate the same landmarks as in the figure above. *Bottom*: the Schlemm's canal (*arrow*) location just prior to de-roofing. Note the distance between the canal and the anterior edge of the surgical limbus

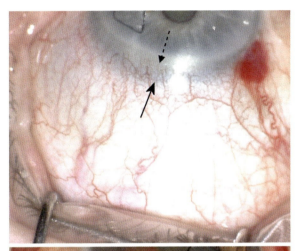
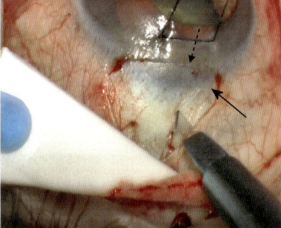
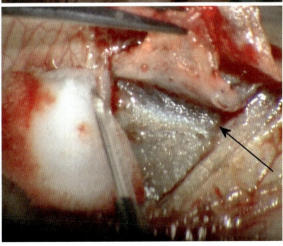

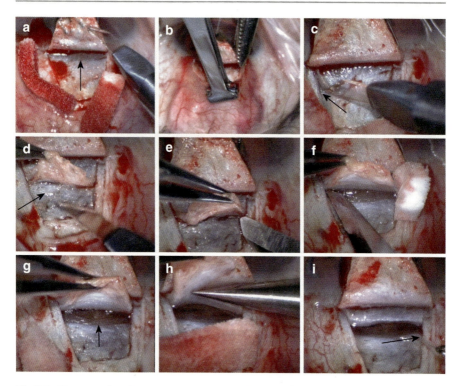

Fig. 3.2 Nonpenetrating glaucoma surgery, creation of the trabeculo-Descemet's filtration membrane. (**a**) *Arrows* indicate dissection of outer sclera flap 1 mm into clear cornea. (**b**) Posterior diffuse MMC application for 1–3 min. (**c**) Deep sclera flap delineation. Edges deepened till Schlemm's canal is cut (*arrow*) and choroid visible at posterior edge. (**d**) The deep sclera fibers (*arrow*) become circumferentially orientated just before the Schlemm's canal is reached. (**e**, **f**) The lateral edges are cut with a No. 11 blade on a Bard-Parker handle. This blade has a blunt tip and posterior edge. The blade is angled at 45° to avoid perforation. (**g**) The dissection is continued at least 1 mm into cornea. The juxtacanalicular trabecular meshwork is delineated clearly (*arrow*). Dissection is done by gently rubbing the membrane with a PVA sponge. Sharp instruments are to be avoided. (**h**) The deep flap is excised (**i**) The juxtacanalicular trabecular meshwork is removed with a blunt-tipped forceps to enhance filtration

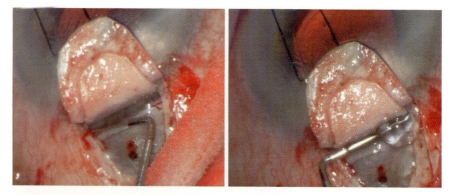

Fig. 3.3 Viscocanalostomy. The Schlemm's canal is dilated by forcefully injecting Healon GV™ through the cut ends

Fig. 3.4 Gonioscopic view of the superior angle after canaloplasty. Iris is partially covering the TDM. The 10/0 prolene suture is clearly seen in the Schlemm's canal

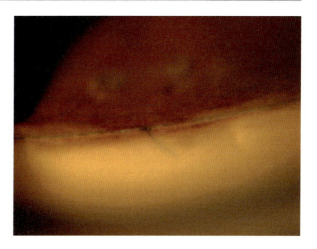

3.3 Efficacy and Outcomes for NPGS

3.3.1 Deep Sclerectomy

In a series of 194 eyes of 160 consecutive patients who had primary phakic DS, the probability of achieving an IOP of less than 19 mmHg without medications or needle revisions was 85 % at 1 year and 78 % at 3 years (Anand et al. 2011). IOP of less than 13 mmHg was achieved without medications or needle revision in 68 % at 1 year and 60 % at 3 years.

In a randomized controlled trial, DS with mitomycin C yielded complete success (defined as IOP ≤21 mmHg without antiglaucoma medications) in 79 % (15/19) of eyes at 1 year and 53 % (10/19) of eyes at 4 years (Cillino et al. 2005, 2008). Qualified success (defined as IOP ≤21 mmHg with or without antiglaucoma medications) was seen in 100 % of eyes at 1 year and 79 % (15/19) of eyes at 4 years.

In another randomized controlled trial, 43 patients were allocated to DS with reticulated hyaluronic acid (SK-GEL) scleral implant and mitomycin C (Russo et al. 2008). No goniopuncture or bleb needling was performed. At 4 years, 51 % of eyes had complete success (defined as achievement of target IOP without antiglaucoma medications) for a target IOP of <21 mmHg, while 33 % of eyes had complete success for a target IOP of <18 mmHg.

Reviews of the literature differ in their conclusions about whether DS offers an equivalent degree of IOP control to trabeculectomy (Eldaly et al. 2014; Rulli et al. 2013).

There is consensus that, compared to DS, trabeculectomy has a higher risk of complications such as hypotony (relative risk (RR) 2.1), choroidal effusion (RR 3.8), cataract (RR 3.3), and shallow anterior chamber (RR 4.1) (Rulli et al. 2013). Blebitis (1 %) and endophthalmitis (0.5 %) have been observed during long-term follow-up of patients who have had DS (Anand et al. 2011).

3.3.2 Viscocanalostomy

In a randomized controlled trial, 35 % of the 25 patients allocated to VC had total success (IOP 6–21 mmHg without medication) at 3 years (Yalvac et al. 2004). Qualified success (IOP 6–21 mmHg with medication) was achieved in 74 % of the patients at 3 years.

Kobayashi et al. (2003) conducted a randomized controlled trial using a paired design in which one eye of each participant received VC whereas the other had trabeculectomy. At 12 months, 64 % of the eyes treated with VC, achieved IOP ≤ 20 mmHg without medication versus 88 % of the eyes treated with trabeculectomy.

Recent systematic reviews and meta-analyses of the available evidence suggest that VC is less effective at controlling IOP than trabeculectomy (Eldaly et al. 2014; Rulli et al. 2013). However, some authors have commented that VC requires a learning curve that may be relevant to outcomes (Eldaly et al. 2014; Mendrinos et al. 2008).

Compared to VC, trabeculectomy has a higher risk of complications such as hypotony (relative risk (RR) 2.6), choroidal effusion (RR 6.0), cataract (RR 3.8), and shallow anterior chamber (RR 5.5) (Rulli et al. 2013).

3.3.3 Canaloplasty

In a prospective series of 94 patients (Lewis et al. 2011), a suture was successfully placed in 74 (79 %) of them. Mean IOP was reduced from 24.7 mmHg at baseline to 15.3 mmHg at 1 year. This result needs to be interpreted with caution because 1-year outcomes were reported for fewer than two-thirds of the patients.

No randomized controlled trials have been conducted to compare canaloplasty with trabeculectomy. In a retrospective, nonrandomized comparative case series, canaloplasty achieved a 32 % reduction in IOP at 12 months compared to 43 % for the trabeculectomy group (Ayyala et al. 2011).

In the series of Lewis et al. (2011), adverse events were reported in 16 %, with hyphema (3 %) and elevated IOP (3 %) being the commonest.

3.4 Complications for NPGS

Nonpenetrating surgery offers a lower rate of complications when compared to conventional trabeculectomy (17 % vs. 65 %, respectively), with or without antimetabolites according to a Cochrane meta-analysis (Eldaly et al. 2014). The presence of the TDM and absence of an iridectomy result in a stable and quiet anterior chamber. The TDM acts as a flow-resistor, preventing shallow anterior chambers and choroidal detachments. However, it is also recognized that with NPGS procedures, surgical learning curve is steeper and that complication rates depend on skill and experience of the surgeon.

Many of the complications found in NPGS overlap with trabeculectomy, which have been covered in the previous chapter. This section will focus on complications specific to DS, VCT, and canaloplasty.

3.4.1 Intraoperative Complications for NPGS

Precise scleral flap dissection is crucial. The outer or superficial scleral flap should be half to third thickness. If too thin, aqueous will transude through the flap. Also a thin scleral flap is prone to necrosis due to a poor vascular supply. This is particularly relevant if MMC or bevacizumab are used (Fig. 3.5).

The inner or deep sclera flap dissection is crucial. If too shallow, the dissection will pass over the SC with little or no filtration. If the dissection is quite shallow with a "white" scleral bed, a third deep flap may be dissected at the correct depth to deroof the SC. If the dissection is slightly shallow and uneven, tissues forming the SC roof can be grasped and avulsed as shown in Fig. 3.6.

Perforation of the TDM is the most common intraoperative complication. The incidence of perforation is around 30 % for the novice and decreases to 2–3 % in the more experienced surgeon (Karlen et al. 1999; Sanchez et al. 1997). Perforation of the TDM can be classified by size into microperforations or large transverse perforation and by location into anterior or posterior.

TDM microperforations often occur while extending the lateral edges of the flap into the cornea. To avoid perforations, the eye should be made soft by releasing aqueous via a paracentesis. This should be done just before the SC is deroofed. If these microperforations are anterior with minimal shallowing of the anterior chamber, the procedure should be continued as normal. Sometimes the microperforation can be left covered by the corneal–scleral stump. The dissection of the TDM should be meticulous and the surgeon should avoid the temptation to complete the operation quickly after an anterior perforation. The outer sclera flap may be suture tightly

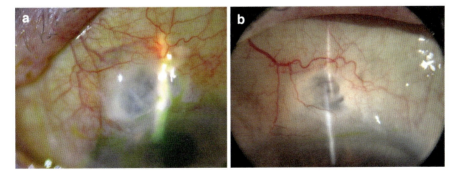

Fig. 3.5 Necrosis of the superficial (outer sclera flap). (**a**) Necrosis and blebitis occurred within the first month after DS with subconjunctival bevacizumab in an 80-year-old Caucasian female with severe Sjogren's syndrome and dry eyes. (**b**) Scleral necrosis observed 2 years after DS with MMC. Patient was asymptomatic and IOP in low teens

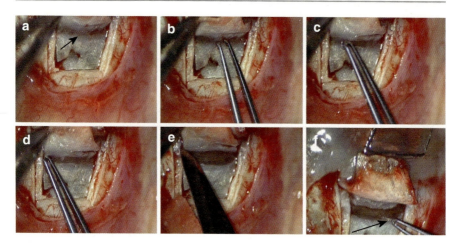

Fig. 3.6 Superficial dissection of the inner scleral flap (**a** and **b**). The scleral flap is placed under tension to tent the scleral fibers overlying the SC and these are grasped with a blunt-tipped forceps and avulsed (**c, d**). The SC is now deroofed with free flow of aqueous and the procedure is continued (**e, f**) The juxtacanalicular tissues are also meticulously removed (*arrow*)

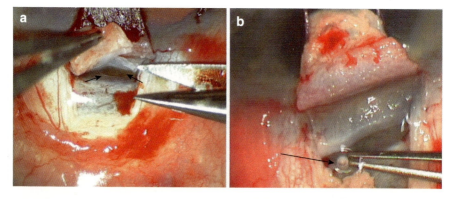

Fig. 3.7 Perforations of the TDM. (**a**) Large transverse perforation (*arrows*) and (**b**) a small posterior perforation while removing JXT tissue with gush of aqueous (*arrow*)

and the anterior chamber reformed at the end of the procedure. The use of viscoelastic to maintain the anterior chamber is to be discouraged as residual viscoelastic may cause a postoperative IOP rise. A large transverse tear at the junction between the trabeculum and Descemet's membrane (corresponds to Schwalbe's line) may occur spontaneously or on minimal applied pressure with a PVA spear (Fig. 3.7). The incidence has not been reported but may occur in 1–2 % of cases. In both a posterior tear and a transverse tear, the iris will relapse and an iridectomy should be performed (Fig. 3.8). The surgeon can excise the deep flap and perform a punch sclerectomy under the superficial flap, converting the procedure to a trabeculectomy. If the deep flap has already been is higher and tight sutures and good closure is imperative. It is advisable to dissect a half-thickness outer sclera flap during the

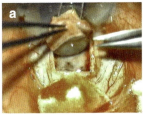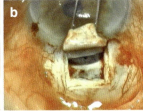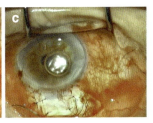

Fig. 3.8 Transverse spontaneous linear perforation with iris prolapse (**a**). The iris was reposited with intradermal intracameral Miochol® and a small peripheral iridectomy was performed (**b**). The inner scleral flap was excised and the outer flap sutured with interrupted 10/0 nylon sutures (**c**). The IOP was 12 mmHg at 3 years after surgery

surgeon's learning curve to ensure watertight closure in case of perforation. Often the transverse linear perforation is not visible on postoperative gonioscopy (Fig. 3.8).

Intraocular bleeding is rare in NPGS because the IOP is reduced slowly and a peripheral iridotomy is not performed. Blood reflux from Schlemm's canal may occur when the episcleral venous pressure rises above the IOP. This may be a favorable sign, indicating an intact outflow pathway. It may fill the subscleral lake and may perhaps stimulate subscleral fibrosis postoperatively. Some experts believe that early laser goniopuncture may be indicated in this situation.

Descemet's membrane detachment (DMD) can occur in all three types of NPGS. The detachment tends to extend from the surgical site in DS and VCT, but tends to occur 180° from the polypropylene suture knot in canaloplasty.

In VCT, the detachment is usually noted at the time of forceful injection of viscoelastic. The management involves removal of the viscoelastic and injection of anterior chamber air bubble tamponade. Rarely, blood can be trapped within the detachment. This blood and can be left if it is peripheral, although it may take months to clear. There is one reported case of blood remnants still visible 2 years after surgery (O'Brart et al. 2004). Hemorrhagic Descemet's detachment involving the visual axis can lead to long-term decrease in visual acuity (Yalvac et al. 2004). Air tamponade is helpful in this situation but occasionally inert gas (such as perfluoropropane (C3F8) or sulfur hexafluoride (SF6) gas), or fixation sutures (descemetopexy) may be needed.

DMD after canaloplasty is not uncommon. In a large case series, DMD was observed 12 out of 124 eyes (7.2 %). Eighty-three percent (10/12) of the DMDs involved the inferior quadrants and measured <3 mm. Hemorrhage within the DMD was seen in 58 %. Two patients had large detachments measuring 5–6 mm extending into the visual axis. DMD resolved completely with or without drainage except for 1 patient who developed corneal decompensation, needing penetrating keratoplasty (Jaramillo et al. 2014).

DMD occurs less frequently after DS. A database search of 1250 DS and combined phacoemulsification and DS procedures done in our institution over 14 years, we identified four cases (0.003 %). Three were observed 2–4 months after DS and

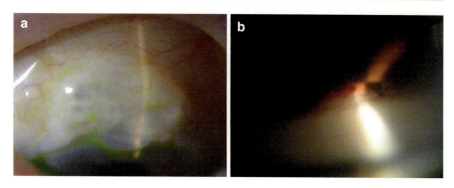

Fig. 3.9 Bleb (**a**) and gonioscopy (**b**) 3 years after DS with subconjunctival bevazizumab and a large transverse perforation. The iris at the lateral edge of the iridectomy is attached to the TDM. However the linear perforation has closed spontaneously

one more than 2 years after surgery (Fig. 3.9). All four eyes had IOP over 20 mmHg. Interestingly, the DMD resolved after laser goniopuncture in one case and after needle revision in three cases (Anand N, unpublished data). The implication is that the etiology of DMD after DS differs from that of VCT. DMD after DS may become manifest if the outflow resistance is high and the aqueous passing through the TDM then accumulates between the corneal stroma and Descemet's membrane. In a case series of nine patients with DMD, four after VCT and five after DS, the authors have emphasized this difference. DMD after VCT is observed immediately after surgery and weeks to month after DS. They performed descemetopexy in four eyes (Ravinet et al. 2002).

Intraoperative adverse events specific to canaloplasty include the inability to cannulate the Schlemm's canal, trauma to the canal and microcatheter passage into the suprachoroidal space (Grieshaber et al. 2011). Difficulties in cannulating Schlemm's canal is usually related to the dissection, identification and de-roofing of the canal. Resistance or blockage of the microcatheter may occur due to a tight opening, hitting an open collector channel, an incomplete canal or scarring in the canal. Injection of viscoelastic into the canal can aid penetration, by dilation and lubrication. The surgeon can also try passing the microcatheter in the opposite direction. Excess force may cause a tear in the trabecular meshwork and cause microcatheter penetration into the anterior chamber. The polypropylene suture is passed through the canal and tightened to maintain its patency. If the suture breaks during knot-tying, then it will need to be replaced. In case of unsuccessful circumferential SC catheterization, the procedure may be converted into 180° metal trabeculotomy. If the tension suture cheese wires through the trabecular meshwork after successful complete catheterization, it is converted into 360° trabeculotomy (Alnahrawy et al. 2015).

Precise suturing of the conjunctival flap is not so critical after NPGS procedures. There is very little flow into the subconjunctival space after VCT and a slow flow after DS. Conjunctival buttonholing and retraction likewise do not have the serious implications as after trabeculectomy.

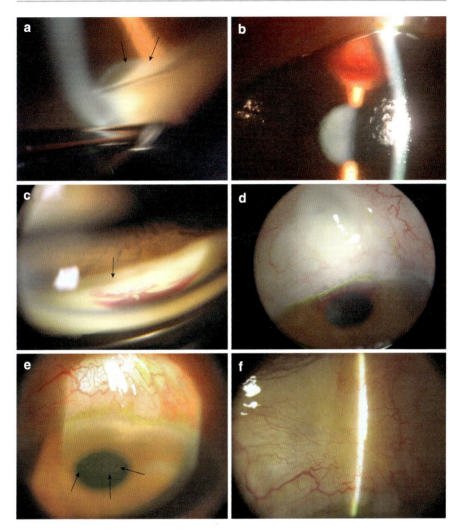

Fig. 3.10 (**a**) A 76-year-old Caucasian male was seen in clinic with IOP of 21 mmHg and a detachment of the Descemet's membrane (*arrows*). (**b**) Needle revision was done with subconjunctival MMC 0.02 mg. Blood filled the space between the DM and corneal stroma (*arrows*). (**c**) Three months later, there was still some blood but with no contiguity with the trabeculo-Descemet's window (*arrows*) and subscleral lake. The bleb was cystic. (**d**) A year later (**e, f**), the IOP had increased to 25 mmHg and the bleb had failed. The faint outline of the DM detachment could still be seen (*arrows*)

3.4.2   Early Postoperative Complications for NPGS

A meta-analysis on prospective comparative studies of NPGS and trabeculectomy concluded that the absolute risk of hypotony, choroidal effusion, cataract, and flat or shallow anterior chamber was higher after trabeculectomy (Rulli et al.).

This is explained by the presence of an additional level of resistance, the TDM. Early complications differ slightly between DS and VCT and canaloplasty. Early hypotony is desirable after DS as the outer scleral flap is sutured loosely to allow subconjunctival aqueous outflow and has been considered to be a favorable prognostic indicator (Shaarawy et al. 2004). In VCT and canaloplasty, the outer scleral flap is tightly sutured, the IOP is between 10 and 20 mmHg and some authors have gone to the extent of reporting a subconjunctival bleb as a complication after VCT.

Early bleb-related complications, such as conjunctival edge leaks and overexuberant blebs with dysesthesia, though uncommon, may be seen after DS. Early conjunctival edge leaks invariably resolve in 1–2 weeks even if MMC has been used with DS and may need resuturing only if the procedure was complicated by intraoperative perforation (Anand et al. 2011).

Hyphema is uncommon after DS (2–15 %) and is due to low early postoperative IOP and blood reflux into the SC (Anand et al. 2011; Kozobolis et al. 2002). Hyphema occurs more frequently after VCT and canaloplasty as there is more trauma with microperforations to the inner wall of the SC. According to one study, hyphema (average height 1.8 mm) may be quite common after canaloplasty, can be seen in 85 % and usually resolves after a week. IOP < 16 mmHg without medications depended significantly on the presence of hyphema. The authors felt that it possibly represented a restored and patent physiologic aqueous outflow system (Grieshaber et al. 2013). Blood in subscleral space above the TDM is occasionally observed in the early postoperative period. It may stimulate fibrosis and lead to early failure. If it persists for than 2–3 weeks and the IOP is high, laser goniopuncture may be considered (Barnebey 2013).

The IOP may be high the early postoperative period after VCT and may sometimes be due to retained viscoelastic. This can be managed by topical antihypotensive agents. Gonioscopy is essential if the IOP is elevated immediately after surgery. The TDM maybe occluded by the iris. This may rarely happen even after an uncomplicated procedure. The mechanism may be a low IOP and a higher posterior chamber pressure pushing the iris towards the TDM. Eyes with a high plateau iris are susceptible. Management is Argon and/or Nd:YAG laser iridoplasty or surgical revision as described in the section for laser goniopuncture.

3.4.3 Late Postoperative Complications for NPGS

There are few delayed complications after nonaugmented NPGS. Most delayed complications are due to intraoperative perforation, laser goniopuncture and adjunctive MMC. Direct trauma to the eye can cause rupture of the TDM with iris prolapsed (Fig. 3.11). This is extremely rare and related to the severity of the force applied to the eye. The TDM can withstand high IOPs.

Bleb-related complications include fibrosis and encapsulation. The conjunctival filtering bleb is generally very shallow and diffuse. Needle revision of the fibrosed bleb can be performed, like after trabeculectomy. It is usually performed after laser

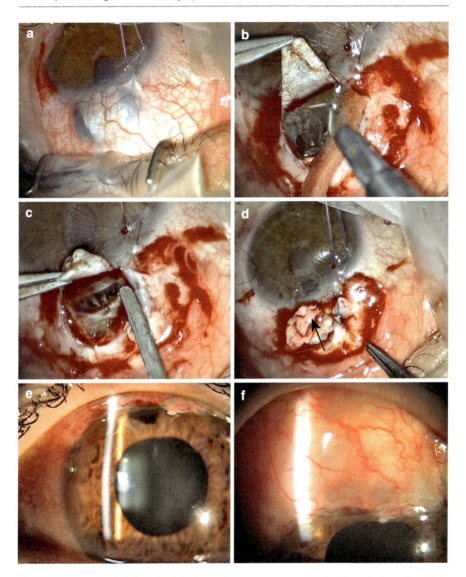

Fig. 3.11 (**a**) Caucasian female with direct trauma to eye presented with peaked pupil and iris prolapse through the membrane and was visible under the conjunctiva. The surgical site was explored and the prolapsed iris was excised (**b, c**). Tenon's capsule was sutured over scleral flap to decrease leak through the thin superficial scleral flap (**d**). The patient had no postoperative complications with a deep anterior chamber and good bleb a week after the revision (**e, f**)

goniopuncture and MMC is the preferred antifibrotic agent. The probability of maintaining IOP less than 19 mmHg without glaucoma medications is about 50 % 5 years after needle revision of DS. Needle revision has significant risks and complications including iris incarceration, bleb leaks, infections and hypotony (Koukkoulli et al. 2015). Needle revision of encapsulated blebs after DS has been reported but no long-term outcomes are available. Like trabeculectomy, there is a probably a high rate of recurrence of encapsulation or failure.

The incidence of surgically induced cataract is low. Decrease in visual acuity due to cataract formation is more common in trabeculectomy compared to NPGS (Eldaly et al. 2014). In head-to-head studies, Russo et al. reported 9/50 developed cataracts in the trabeculectomy group compared to 2/43 in the NPGS group (Russo et al. 2008). Yalvac reported 7/25 and 2/25 respectively, while Kobayashi reported 2/25 and 0/25 respectively (Kobayashi et al. 2003; Yalvac et al. 2004). The Advanced Glaucoma Intervention Study (AIGS) estimated that the rate of cataract formation after the first trabeculectomy was 78 % at 5 years. The risk of cataract is doubled if there is a significant postoperative inflammation or a flat anterior chamber which is rare after NPGS (AGIS Investigators 2001).

The probability of cataract surgery after DS is 2.5 % at 1 year, 16.4 % at 3 years, 26 % at 5 years, and 38 % at 7 years. The median survival time (50 % probability) for cataract surgery after DS was 155 months. Age was the most significant risk factor. MMC application at time of DS was not significantly associated with cataract surgery. However, 26 % of eyes needed an increase in number of glaucoma medications, bleb needling, or further glaucoma surgery to maintain IOP control after phacoemulsification. This is probably due to bleb failure in some eyes, not unlike that seen in trabeculectomy (Anand et al., Poster, American Academy of Ophthalmology, Annual Meeting 2014).

3.5   Complications Specific to Mitomycin C (MMC) Use in NPGS

Subconjunctival MMC application with NPGS will result in a higher frequency of large, avascular and cystic blebs. The reported incidence however varies significantly (Anand and Atherly 2005). Kozobolis et al. reported no avascular cystic blebs in their prospective comparative trial on MMC with DS. They did not do laser goniopuncture and 70 % of blebs had failed by 3 years in both groups. Anand et al. in a retrospective case series observed cystic blebs in 36.5 % of cases. The frequency of cystic blebs was 58 % when MMC was applied on the anterior sclera, and was significantly lower at 30 % when MMC was applied posteriorly with conjunctival edge-protection. Most (60 %) of the eyes had laser goniopuncture and about 15 % had needle revision in the 4-year follow-up. This difference in approach may explain the marked difference in the incidence of avascular blebs reported in the two studies.

There have been two reports of blebitis after DS (Wallin and Montan 2007; Anand et al. 2011) and one report of endophthalmitis (Fig. 3.12) following DS with MMC where intraoperative perforation had occurred (Anand et al. 2011).

MMC is not commonly used with VCT or canaloplasty as these procedures do not rely on subconjunctival drainage. Most authors recommend four to seven sutures to tightly close the scleral flap until no aqueous leakage is seen. With this technique, a postoperative bleb is only found in 0–16 % of cases (Carassa et al. 2003; Sunaric-Megevand and Leuenberger 2001; Stegmann et al. 1999). If two to three sutures are

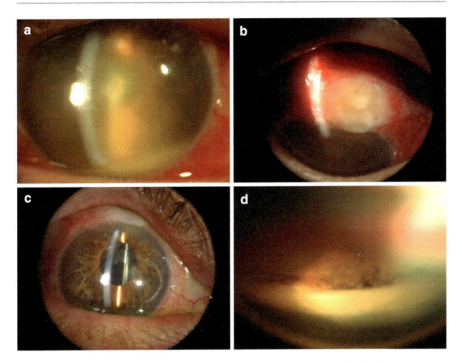

Fig. 3.12 Caucasian female patient with endophthalmitis 2 years after DS with MMC and intraoperative perforation. Three days after intravitreal injection broad-spectrum antibiotics, the hypopyon (**a**) and abscess in the avascular bleb (**b**) can still be seen. The eye improved rapidly (**c**) and gonioscopy at 3 weeks showed iris synechiae (**d**)

used to close the scleral flap, then a bleb is seen more often (57–100 %) (O'Brart et al. 2004; Luke et al. 2002). In a retrospective comparative study of VCT, avascular blebs were observed more frequently, when MMC was applied under the superficial scleral flap (Yarangümeli et al. 2005). In a case series of canaloplasty, MMC was applied under the outer scleral flap before deep flap dissection. Seven eyes (35.0 %) had biomicroscopic evidence of mild conjunctival elevation over the area of incision at 12 months with no complications (Barnebey 2013).

3.6 Laser Procedure After NPGS Goniopuncture

3.6.1 Introduction

NPGS procedures like DS have two levels of resistance to aqueous outflow – the TDM and subconjunctival tissues. Aqueous flow across the TDM may decrease in time due to fibrosis on its external interface. Resistance to outflow may also increase due to progressive fibrosis of the subscleral and subconjunctival tissues. Microperforations in the TDM may be created by Nd:YAG laser, thereby increasing aqueous flow and further increasing efficacy. If goniopuncture is required early, dissection of the TDM may have been inadequate resulting in a thick membrane that yields insufficient rate of filtration (Mendrinos et al. 2008). It may be performed weeks to years after NPGS (Mermoud et al. 1999). Anecdotally laser goniopuncture (LGP) is more effective in lowering IOP in the presence of a subconjunctival filtration bleb. The presence of a bleb with raised IOP implies increasing resistance at the TDM level. More than half the eyes undergoing DS will have laser goniopuncture by 3 years after surgery (Anand and Pilling 2010). DS may be regarded as a two-staged procedure where the TDM is punctured to achieve the target IOP, a few months after the initial surgery.

3.6.2   Procedure

LGP is performed with the Q-switch Nd:YAG laser. A Magnaview™ gonioscopy lens is preferred because of the magnification (×1.3–1.5) and superior view of the angle. The TDM is seen as a semi-transparent diaphanous membrane. The aim is to create a small perforation at the anterior edge of the TDM. Iris may occasionally occlude single central goniopuncture and cover the rest of the TDM. Therefore it is preferable to puncture the TDM at either end. Laser energy levels vary between 2 and 4 mJ, depending on TDM thickness. The TDM may have a concave configuration and the bleb may be quite low before LGP. LGP will allow aqueous to pass through, changing the TDM configuration to convex and increase the height of bleb (Fig. 3.13). Figure 3.14 shows the different varieties of ostia seen after LGP. Prophylactic argon iridoplasty may be performed prior to LGP in eyes with convex peripheral iris or a plateau iris configuration. It may also be indicated in eyes where the TDM is antero-posteriorly narrow.

3.6.3   Efficacy and Outcomes

LGP can be done after all three types of NPGS. It is perhaps most effective after DS as the procedure results in the lowest distal resistance to outflow due to the formation of a subconjunctival bleb.

In a large case series of patients who had DS, at 2 years after goniopuncture the probability of maintaining IOP < 15 mmHg with a 20 % decrease from pre-laser IOP and no further glaucoma procedure or medication was 50 % (Anand and Pilling 2010). A similar long-term success rate was reported recently by another study (Al Obeidan 2015).

In a small case series of VCT, 36 % of eyes underwent LGP. Success after LGP, defined as IOP < 19 mm Hg without medication was noted in 33 % by last follow-up (Alp et al. 2010). Grieshaber et al., in a small case series of canaloplasty, performed LGP in 18 % of eyes within 3 months after surgery. They reported a mean IOP drop of 6 mmHg after LGP. Long-term results are not available.

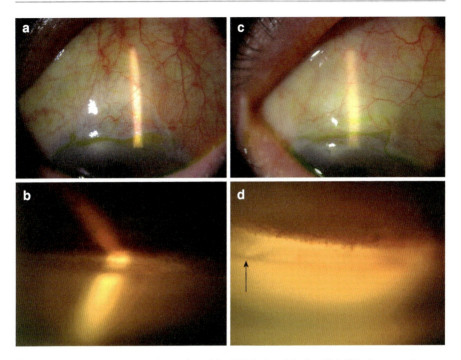

Fig. 3.13 Note the concave configuration of the TDM (**a**) and the low bleb (**b**) prior to goniopuncture. One month after LGP, the bleb is more diffuse (**c**) and the conjunctival vessels are of a smaller caliber due to tissue turgor. The TDM is not convex (**d**) and a small puncture can be seen (*arrow*)

3.6.4   Complications of Laser Goniopuncture

Laser goniopuncture can cause a rapid drop in IOP to leading to iris incarceration. The pressure in the posterior chamber can be higher than in the anterior chamber immediately after LGP, driving the iris into the puncture. This is why most authors advise delaying goniopuncture until at least 3–4 weeks after surgery when sufficient healing has occurred. Hypotony occurs in 0–4 %, and can be associated with choroidal detachment and maculopathy (Mermoud et al. 1999; Anand and Pilling 2010; Vuori 2003). If the IOP is very high, it should be pre-treated with medication to lower the IOP before GP to reduce the pressure differential.

Iris incarceration occurs in around 0–13 % after GP (Vuori 2003; Anand and Pilling 2010; Mermoud et al. 1999). In a case series of 258 patients, the commonest complication of goniopuncture following DS is iris synechiae or incarceration. Overall it was observed in 13 % of cases after LGP. Acute symptomatic rise in IOP occurs in 1.7 % of cases after LGP, due to iris blocking outflow through the TDM. Hypotony has been reported in up to 4 % after goniopuncture, mostly in eyes with adjunctive MMC. Less common complications reported were delayed bleb leak and blebitis. About one in four eyes treated with goniopuncture required argon

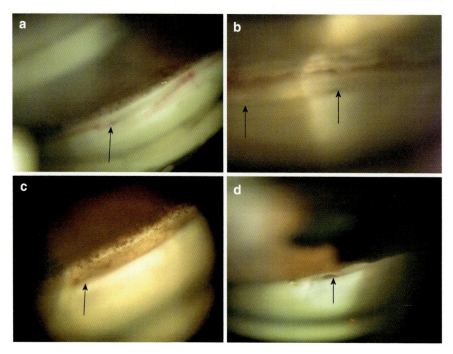

Fig. 3.14 Openings in the TDM (*arrows*) after laser goniopuncture. Blood often refluxes into the Schlemm's canal as the IOP drops below 12 mmHg. (**a**). The gonipunctures should be tiny and barely visible (**b**). A large puncture (**c**) or an inadvertent linear rip of the TDM (**d**) increase the risk of iris incarceration

laser iridoplasty, and a similar proportion required needle revision. The argon laser was done either prophylactically or to remove iris from the TDM or goniopunctures (Anand and Pilling 2010).

In a study with sequential gonioscopy after DS, Sponsel et al. concluded that risk of failure was associated with narrow gonioscopic angle insertion and synechia, but not with shallow approach or trabecular pigmentation (Sponsel et al. 2013). The first intervention for raised IOP and iris synechia or prolapse though perforation or puncture should be Argon and/or Nd:YAG Laser iridoplasty. After instilling a drop of pilocarpine 2 %, Argon laser burns should be used to shrink the iris and pull it away the Descemet's window. The parameters are 100 µm spot size, 0.4–0.5 ms and energy levels between 200 and 500 mW to create microcavitation (bubbles). Nd:YAG laser 1–2 mJ may then be used to disrupt the iris plug or break the synechiae. Sometimes only the latter is needed (Anand and Pilling 2010). If this fails, then surgical release may be necessary via a paracentesis combined with peripheral iridectomy. Focal iridectomy can be performed bimanually via paracenteses using retinal forceps and microscissors in instances of irreducible iris incarceration into the drainage zone (Sponsel et al. 2013).

In order to minimize the risk for iris incarceration, Anand and Pilling recommended the following measures:

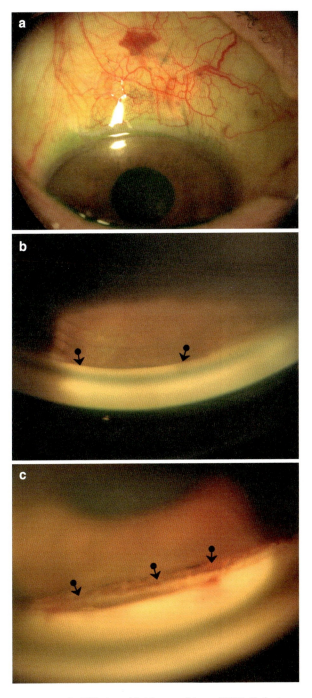

Fig. 3.15 Acute symptomatic IOP rise with iris synechiae at TDM. Patient present with severe pain in eye and an IOP over 50 mmHg 3 months after laser goniopuncture. The bleb was flat and injected (**a**) and the TDM was completely covered by TDM (*arrows* **b**). The iris was removed from the TDM by Argon laser burns (*arrows*, **c**)

- DS is not routinely performed in phakic eyes with shallow anterior chambers and a convex peripheral iris configuration or a high plateau iris configuration.
- During surgery try to make a wide trabeculo-Descemet's membrane window, more than 2 mm.
- Laser goniopuncture is avoided in the first month when the outflow resistance at the subconjunctival level is low.
- Laser puncture is performed at the anterior edge of the TDM, starting with lower energy levels (2–3 mJ) to avoid a large puncture.
- Laser puncture is performed at each lateral edge rather than at the center of the trabeculo-Descemet's membrane window.
- Prophylactic argon iridoplasty is performed where it is felt that the iris may incarcerate in the puncture site and if immediate post-LGP gonioscopy shows contact between the iris and the trabeculo-Descemet's membrane window.
- All patients undergo routine gonioscopy at each follow-up visit to identify any iris incarceration. If not possible, do gonioscopy in all eyes with raised IOP.

References

Al Obeidan SA. Incidence, efficacy and safety of YAG laser goniopuncture following nonpenetrating deep sclerectomy at a university hospital in Riyadh, Saudi Arabia. Saudi J Ophthalmol. 2015;29:95–102.

Alnahrawy O, Blumenstock G, Ziemssen F, Szurman P, Leitritz MA, Dimopoulos S, Voykov B. Exit strategies in canaloplasty: intraoperative conversion into 180-degree trabeculotomy or 360-degree trabeculotomy in cases of unsuccessful catheterisation of Schlemm's canal: influence of degree of canal cleavage. Graefes Arch Clin Exp Ophthalmol. 2015;253(5):779–84. doi: 10.1007/s00417-015-2955-9. Epub 2015 Feb 18.

Alp MN, Yarangumeli A, Koz OG, Kural G. Nd:YAG laser goniopuncture in viscocanalostomy: penetration in non-penetrating glaucoma surgery. Int Ophthalmol. 2010;30(3):245–52. doi:10.1007/s10792-009-9312-0.

Anand N, Atherley C. Deep sclerectomy augmented with mitomycin C. Eye (Lond). 2005;19(4):442–50. doi:10.1038/sj.eye.6701403.

Anand N, Bong C. Deep sclerectomy with bevacizumab and mitomycin C: a comparative study. J Glaucoma. 2015;24(1):25–31. doi:10.1097/IJG.0b013e3182883c0c.

Anand N, Pilling R. Nd:YAG laser goniopuncture after deep sclerectomy: outcomes. Acta Ophthalmol. 2010;88(1):110–5. doi:10.1111/j.1755-3768.2008.01494.x.

Anand N, Kumar A, Gupta A. Primary phakic deep sclerectomy augmented with mitomycin C: long-term outcomes. J Glaucoma. 2011;20(1):21–7. doi:10.1097/IJG.0b013e3181ccb926.

Ayyala RS, Chaudhry AL, Okogbaa CB, et al. Comparison of surgical outcomes between canaloplasty and trabeculectomy at 12 months' follow-up. Ophthalmology. 2011;118:2427–33.

Barnebey HS. Canaloplasty with intraoperative low dosage mitomycin C: a retrospective case series. J Glaucoma. 2013;22(3):201–4. doi:10.1097/IJG.0b013e31824083fb.

Carassa RG, Bettin P, Fiori M, Brancato R. Viscocanalostomy versus trabeculectomy in white adults affected by open-angle glaucoma: a 2-year randomized, controlled trial. Ophthalmology. 2003;110(5):882–7. doi:10.1016/S0161-6420(03)00081-2.

Cillino S, Di Pace F, Casuccio A, et al. Deep sclerectomy versus punch trabeculectomy: effect of low-dosage mitomycin C. Ophthalmologica. 2005;219:281–6.

Cillino S, Di Pace F, Casuccio A, et al. Deep sclerectomy versus trabeculectomy with low-dosage mitomycin C: four-year follow-up. Ophthalmologica. 2008;222:81–7.

Eldaly MA, Bunce C, Elsheikha OZ, Wormald R. Non-penetrating filtration surgery versus tra-beculectomy for open-angle glaucoma. Cochrane Database Syst Rev. 2014;2:CD007059. doi:10.1002/14651858.CD007059.pub2.

Grieshaber MC, Fraenkl S, Schoetzau A, Flammer J, Orgül S. Circumferential viscocanalostomy and suture canal distension (canaloplasty) for whites with open-angle glaucoma. J Glaucoma. 2011;20(5):298–302. doi:10.1097/IJG.0b013e3181e3d46e.

Grieshaber MC, Schoetzau A, Flammer J. Orgül SPostoperative microhyphema as a positive prognostic indicator in canaloplasty. Acta Ophthalmol. 2013;91(2):151–6. doi:10.1111/j.1755-3768.2011.02293.x. Epub 2011 Dec 9

The Advanced Glaucoma Intervention Study (AGIS): 7. The relationship between control of intraocular pressure and visual field deterioration.The AGIS Investigators. Am J Ophthalmol. 2000;130(4):429–40.

Jaramillo A, Foreman J, Ayyala RS. Descemet membrane detachment after canaloplasty: inci-dence and management. J Glaucoma. 2014;23(6):351–4. doi:10.1097/IJG.0b013e318279ca7f.

Karlen ME, Sanchez E, Schnyder CC, Sickenberg M, Mermoud A. Deep sclerectomy with col-lagen implant: medium term results. Br J Ophthalmol. 1999;83(1):6–11.

Kobayashi H, Kobayashi K, Okinami S. A comparison of the intraocular pressure-lowering effect and safety of viscocanalostomy and trabeculectomy with mitomycin C in bilateral open-angle glaucoma. Graefes Arch Clin Exp Ophthalmol. 2003;241(5):359–66. doi:10.1007/s00417-003-0652-6.

Koukkoulli A, Musa F, Anand N. Long-term outcomes of needle revision of failing deep scle-rectomy blebs. Graefes Arch Clin Exp Ophthalmol. 2015;253(1):99–106. doi:10.1007/s00417-014-2810-4.

Kozobolis VP, Christodoulakis EV, Tzanakis N, Zacharopoulos I, Pallikaris IG. Primary deep scle-rectomy versus primary deep sclerectomy with the use of mitomycin C in primary open-angle glaucoma. J Glaucoma. 2002;11(4):287–93.

Krasnov MM. Externalization of Schlemm's canal (sinusotomy) in glaucoma. Br J Ophthalmol. 1968;52(2):157–61.

Lewis RA, von Wolff K, Tetz M, Koerber N, Kearney JR, Shingleton BJ, Samuelson TW. Canaloplasty: three-year results of circumferential viscodilation and tensioning of Schlemm canal using a microcatheter to treat open-angle glaucoma. J Cataract Refract Surg. 2011;37(4):682–90. doi:10.1016/j.jcrs.2010.10.055.

Luke C, Dietlein TS, Jacobi PC, Konen W, Krieglstein GK. A prospective randomized trial of viscocanalostomy versus trabeculectomy in open-angle glaucoma: a 1-year follow-up study. J Glaucoma. 2002;11(4):294–9.

Mendrinos E, Mermoud A, Shaarawy T. Nonpenetrating glaucoma surgery. Surv Ophthalmol. 2008;53:592–630.

Mermoud A, Karlen ME, Schnyder CC, Sickenberg M, Chiou AG, Hediguer SE, Sanchez E. Nd:Yag goniopuncture after deep sclerectomy with collagen implant. Ophthalmic Surg Lasers. 1999;30(2):120–5.

O'Brart DP, Shiew M, Edmunds B. A randomised, prospective study comparing trabeculectomy with viscocanalostomy with adjunctive antimetabolite usage for the management of open angle glaucoma uncontrolled by medical therapy. Br J Ophthalmol. 2004;88(8):1012–7. doi:10.1136/bjo.2003.037432.

Ravinet E, Tritten JJ, Roy S, Gianoli F, Wolfensberger T, Schnyder C, Mermoud A. Descemet membrane detachment after nonpenetrating filtering surgery. J Glaucoma. 2002;11(3):244–52.

Rulli E, Biagioli E, Riva I, et al. Efficacy and safety of trabeculectomy vs nonpenetrating surgical procedures: a systematic review and meta-analysis. JAMA Ophthalmol. 2013;131:1573–82.

Russo V, Scott IU, Stella A, Balducci F, Cosma A, Barone A, Delle Noci N. Nonpenetrating deep sclerectomy with reticulated hyaluronic acid implant versus punch trabeculectomy: a prospec-tive clinical trial. Eur J Ophthalmol. 2008;18(5):751–7.

Sanchez E, Schnyder CC, Mermoud A. Comparative results of deep sclerectomy transformed to trabeculectomy and classical trabeculectomy. Klin Monatsbl Augenheilkd. 1997;210(5):261–4. doi:10.1055/s-2008-1035050.

Shaarawy T, Flammer J, Smits G, Mermoud A. Low first postoperative day intraocular pressure as a positive prognostic indicator in deep sclerectomy. Br J Ophthalmol. 2004;88(5):658–61.

Stegmann RC. Visco-canalostomy: a new surgical technique for open angle glaucoma. An Inst Barraquer. 1995;25:229–32.

Stegmann R, Pienaar A, Miller D. Viscocanalostomy for open-angle glaucoma in black African patients. J Cataract Refract Surg. 1999;25(3):316–22.

Sponsel WE1, Groth SL. Mitomycin-augmented non-penetrating deep sclerectomy: preoperative gonioscopy and postoperative perimetric, tonometric and medication trends. Br J Ophthalmol. 2013;97(3):357–61. doi: 10.1136/bjophthalmol-2012-301886. Epub 2012 Nov 2.

Sunaric-Megevand G, Leuenberger PM. Results of viscocanalostomy for primary open-angle glaucoma. Am J Ophthalmol. 2001;132(2):221–8.

Tamm ER, Carassa RG, Albert DM, Gabelt BT, Patel S, Rasmussen CA, Kaufman PL. Viscocanalostomy in rhesus monkeys. Arch Ophthalmol. 2004 Dec;122(12):1826–38.

Vuori ML. Complications of Neodymium:YAG laser goniopuncture after deep sclerectomy. Acta Ophthalmol Scand. 2003;81(6):573–6.

Wallin OJ, Montan PG. Blebitis after deep sclerectomy. Eye (Lond). 2007;21(2):258–60. doi:10.1038/sj.eye.6702494.

Yalvac IS, Sahin M, Eksioglu U, Midillioglu IK, Aslan BS, Duman S. Primary viscocanalostomy versus trabeculectomy for primary open-angle glaucoma: three-year prospective randomized clinical trial. J Cataract Refract Surg. 2004;30(10):2050–7. doi:10.1016/j.jcrs.2004.02.073.

Yarangümeli A, Köz OG, Alp MN, Elhan AH, Kural G. Viscocanalostomy with mitomycin-C: a preliminary study. Eur J Ophthalmol. 2005;15(2):202–8.

Zimmerman TJ, Kooner KS, Ford VJ, Olander KW, Mandlekorn RM, Rawlings EF, Leader BJ, Koskan AJ. Trabeculectomy vs. nonpenetrating trabeculectomy: a retrospective study of two procedures in phakic patients with glaucoma. Ophthalmic Surg. 1984;15(9):734–40.

Trabeculectomy

4

Rashmi G. Mathew and Ian E. Murdoch

If you have not seen all the complications mentioned in this chapter, the likelihood is, you have not operated enough. Every surgeon has complications. What makes an excellent surgeon is the ability to deal with the complication safely and appropriately. Most of the complications outlined below are fortunately rare and little or no evidence exists for their management. Much of what is written below is from our own personal experience.

A key factor to the success of any operation is careful preoperative assessment and planning. Prevention is better than cure. Anticipation of potential problems prior to surgery enables a surgeon to take precautions to minimize the likelihood of complications and be prepared, should they arise. Careful preoperative assessment of the patient and risk factors also allows the patient to be counseled appropriately in the face of increased risks and have an appropriate level of expectation regarding the surgery. As with all surgeries, each step needs to be meticulously performed in order to garner the best possible outcome.

In this chapter we look at important preoperative, perioperative, early and late postoperative factors in turn. For each, we present a largely personal view for consideration, looking at tips to prevent as well as manage complications of trabeculectomy surgery. The trabeculectomy technique we use is a version of the "Moorfields Safe Surgery" technique (Dhingra and Khaw 2009). A fornix-based, conjunctival flap, followed by the application of cytotoxic on sponges to a broad sub-Tenon's space extending behind the posterior edge of the anticipated sclera flap in an

R.G. Mathew (✉)
Department of Glaucoma, Moorfields Eye Hospital NHSFT, London, UK

Honorary Clinical Senior Lecturer, Centre for Medical Education, Institute of Health Sciences Education, Barts and the London School of Medicine at Queen Mary, University of London, London, UK
e-mail: rashmi.mathew@moorfields.nhs.uk

I.E. Murdoch
Institute of Ophthalmology, University College, London, London, UK

Moorfields Eye Hospital NHS Foundation Trust, London, UK

F. Carbonaro, K. Sheng Lim (eds.), *Managing Complications in Glaucoma Surgery*, DOI 10.1007/978-3-319-49416-6_4, © Springer International Publishing AG 2017 outward fan. Copious washout of the cytotoxic is followed by creation of a rectangular scleral flap, paracentesis, sclerostomy, and peripheral iridectomy. Releasable 10/0 nylon sutures are used to close the sclera flap and interrupted 10/0 nylon sutures to secure the Tenon and conjunctiva to the limbus.

4.1 Preoperative Risk Factors

4.1.1 Ocular Factors

Risk Factor Refractive Error: High myopia.
  High myopes tend to have more elastic sclera and may also have thinner sclera.

Potential Complication Hypotony.

How to Avoid We recommend using a minimum of three releasable sutures for the closure of the trabeculectomy flap on table. Check for any leaks on the table with 2 % fluorescein after tying of the releasables. If leaks are present on the table, tighten the existing releasables and reassess with 2 % fluorescein. Should the leak persist, use further releasables or fixed sutures depending on the location of the leak.
  The other key to avoiding hypotony in these patients is the creation of a relatively thick flap and avoidance of a thin flap. Water tight closure in thin flaps is difficult and sutures may cheese-wire the flap.
  It is also important that these patients wear their eye shield while sleeping and avoid heavy lifting, bending, and eye rubbing in the early postoperative period.

Risk Factor Refractive Error: High hypermetropia.

Potential Complication Aqueous misdirection.

How to Avoid Avoidance of hypotony and anterior chamber shallowing is the key. We recommend a minimum of three releasables to close the trabeculectomy flap. Always check for any leaks on the table with 2 % fluorescein. At the end of the operation instill a drop of 1 % atropine and continue this once daily for at least 4 weeks. It is also important that these patients wear their eye shield while sleeping and avoid heavy lifting, bending, and eye rubbing in the early postoperative period.

Risk Factor Ocular surgery: coexistence of cataract.

Potential Complication Aggressive postoperative wound healing.

How to Avoid The question about whether to perform cataract surgery before or after trabeculectomy surgery is an old chestnut and is widely debated in glaucoma circles. The literature reports between 10 and 61 % of trabeculectomies failing after cataract surgery (Mathew and Murdoch 2011; Chen et al. 1998; Swamynathan et al.

2004; Crichton and Kirker 2001; Rebolleda and Munoz-Negrete 2002; Park et al. 1997; Casson et al. 2002; Wong et al. 2009; Ehnrooth et al. 2005). Interpretation of the results is, however, hampered by very few having a control group, different study methods, definitions of failure, and patient groups. To our knowledge there are only two case–control studies in the literature comparing the eyes that had trabeculectomy alone with those that had trabeculectomy with subsequent cataract surgery. One study showed no difference in failure rates at 1 year (Chen et al. 1998) and the other showed a significantly higher failure rate in the group that had cataract extraction subsequent to trabeculectomy surgery (Swamynathan et al. 2004). It has been shown that flare exists in the anterior chamber for up to 6 months after cataract surgery (Siriwardena et al. 2000). In comparison, anterior chamber flare levels return to base-line levels 4 weeks after trabeculectomy surgery. This can have implications for the success of trabeculectomy surgery and whether to perform cataract surgery before or after trabeculectomy, if cataract is present. The debate is still unresolved and we recommend full discussion with your patient of the pros and cons of the three options of cataract surgery first, trabeculectomy first, or combined surgery. Factors such as severity of glaucoma, severity of cataract, time constraints, social circumstance, state of fellow eye, and expectations all need to be considered.

Risk Factor Previous ocular surgery: vitrectomized eye, corneal graft surgery, aphakia, conjunctival scarring, squint surgery.

Potential Complication Difficult conjunctival dissection and aggressive wound healing.

How to Avoid It is important to carefully plan surgery in these cases and a number of factors need to be considered. It is thought that the Tenon's fibroblasts are acti-vated from previous surgery and these patients often have a tendency to mount an aggressive wound healing response for this reason. An important consideration is careful assessment of the mobility of the conjunctiva, as this may be tethered down in places from previous surgery, making clean dissection difficult. One surgical tip is to use a 30-gauge needle with saline to hydrodissect under the conjunctiva, sepa-rating it from the sclera to facilitate trauma free dissection. If there has been previ-ous vitreo-retinal surgery, it is important to assess for the presence of retinal buckles. Aqueous shunt surgery is often first line for these patients. The plate can often be placed behind the buckle and the tube can run over the buckle or a small area of buckle can be removed to allow the tube to lie flat. One must bear in mind that the sclera under the buckle can often be very thin and in extreme cases may warrant a scleral patch graft to restore scleral integrity.

Risk Factor Adverse ocular surface Stevens–Johnson syndrome, ocular cicatricial pemphigoid, atopic keratoconjunctivitis, drop intolerances (chronic red eye), blepharitis.

Potential Complication Excessive scarring, infection.

How to Avoid The commonest of these conditions is drop intolerance and chronic red eye as a result. These eyes are prone to scarring and it is important to optimize the ocular environment prior to embarking upon surgery.

Patients with drop allergies or intolerance to preservatives might benefit from a switch to preservative-free preparations. Consider giving them a "drop holiday" by stopping all topical medication and lowering the intraocular pressure with oral acet-azolamide on a short-term basis if not medically contraindicated. It is important to check that they do not have renal impairment and ensure that their serum potassium is regularly monitored, as it can cause hypokalemia. On commencement of acet-azolamide, advise patients to take the tablets on a full stomach and increase their intake of potassium-rich foods, such as bananas and tomatoes.

One may also consider the use of short-term preoperative steroid drops prior to surgery. This has been shown to reduce the number of fibroblasts and inflammatory cells present within the conjunctiva (Broadway et al. 1996).

For those with blepharitis (especially posterior blepharitis (Poornima Rai, Personal communication)) it is very important to detect and treat the blepharitis with appropriate therapy including good lid hygiene, topical fusidic acid, or oral tetracyclines.

In all cases with chronic disturbance of the ocular surface consider aqueous shunt surgery.

Risk Factor Compromised lacrimal system (chronic dacrocystitis, mucoceles).

Potential Complication Infection.

How to Avoid In patients with chronic dacrocystitis and mucoceles, the patient is predisposed to bleb-related infection and endophthalmitis. It is important to only perform glaucoma surgery once the patient has had this definitively treated, most commonly with a dacryocystorhinostomy.

Risk Factor Abnormal vasculature, Sturge–Weber syndrome, caroticocavernous fistula, arterio-venous malformations.

Potential Complication Excessive scarring and failure, excessive intraoperative bleeding.

How to Avoid In those patients with caroticocavernous fistula, Sturge–Weber syndrome, and arterio-venous malformations of the conjunctiva and episclera, it is important to bear in mind that these patients have a propensity to bleed. These patients may also have choroidal hemangiomas and other retinal vascular abnormalities, thus making them more prone to suprachoroidal hemorrhages. In such cases, it may be that aqueous shunt surgery is an alternative to consider.

Risk Factor Lash trichiasis, lid absence.

Potential Complication Exogenous endophthalmitis.

How to Avoid It is important that aberrant lash growth is remedied before undertaking trabeculectomy surgery. The patient may require simple lash electrolysis or plicating procedure to optimize lid position. In cases of partial lid absence, consider aqueous shunt surgery and place in a position, where some lid is present.

Risk Factor Uveitis.

Potential Complication Hypotony posttrabeculectomy surgery.

How to Avoid These patients often have hypotony in the context of a flat bleb. It is often a matter of tiding them over until the ciliary body perks up. It is important to maintain the patient on appropriate therapy for the duration of the inflammatory eye disease. There are two benefits of high-dose topical steroids; ensuring ciliary body function to keep flow through the newly established trabeculectomy and second, reducing the potential for scarring, when little flow or no flow is present through the sclerostomy.

4.1.2 Systemic Factors

Risk Factor Diabetes.

Potential complication(s) Poor wound healing; failure in those with active diabetic retinopathy; postoperative hypotony, due to "brittle" ciliary body function, secondary to ischemia.

How to Avoid Multiple complications may arise in patients with diabetic eye disease. Again, the importance of thorough preoperative assessment and counseling of the patient cannot be stressed enough. Prior to undergoing surgery, blood sugar control must be optimized. In those with poor control and particularly those with active diabetic retinopathy or proliferative retinopathy, an aqueous shunt is usually the first-line surgical approach. This is because VEGF levels in these patients are usually high and can lead to aggressive scarring and failure of trabeculectomy surgery. It is important to work closely with the medical retinal experts ensuring that full laser and medical therapy are undertaken to control the diabetic eye disease. In those with neovascular glaucoma, consider giving anti-VEGF therapy a few days prior to surgery, to initiate regression of neovascularization, limit perioperative bleeding, and reduce pain from ocular ischemia (Kotecha et al. 2011).

Diabetics are also prone to poor wound healing, so ensure that flap closure is water-tight and conjunctival closure is especially secure, as these eyes are much less forgiving.

Diabetic patients can behave like uveitics, due to "brittle" ciliary body function. They may also have hypotony in the context of a flat bleb.

Risk Factor Hypertension, COPD, anticoagulation.

Potential Complication Suprachoroidal hemorrhage.

How to Avoid Suprachoroidal hemorrhage generally occurs secondary to sudden drops in ocular pressure or prolonged periods of hypotony. In a surgical context this is usually on the operating table or the day after surgery. Hypertension and COPD as well as older age are risk factors for suprachoroidal hemorrhage. Anticoagulation, for example with warfarin, is not a confirmed independent risk factor, but can certainly exacerbate a suprachoroidal hemorrhage. For warfarinized patients, ensure the international normalization ratio (INR), is within the therapeutic range prior to surgery. For most procedures, it has been recommended to stop the anticoagulant treatment prior to surgery and then restart within 12–24 h after their surgery, but this should only be done in conjunction with the patient's physician (Kiire et al. 2014).

Both hypertension and COPD should be optimized before surgery and sudden reduction of the intraocular pressure and prolonged periods of hypotony on table should be minimized. As part of our standard trabeculectomy technique, we always create an anterior chamber paracentesis, after fashioning the trabeculectomy flap and prior to creation of the sclerostomy and have balanced salt solution (BSS) ready to hand to refill the anterior chamber, should it shallow. In high risk cases, one may also consider the use of an AC maintainer to avoid sudden AC shallowing and prolonged hypotony. We also recommend considering preplacement of releasables, in order to close the eye and regain integrity as quickly as possible, once the sclerostomy and peripheral iridectomy have been created.

4.2   Perioperative Complications

Risk Factor High intraocular pressure.

Potential complication Decompression retinopathy; suprachoroidal hemorrhage.

How to avoid In patients with uncontrolled intraocular pressure requiring urgent surgery, it is important that their intraocular pressure is optimized as much as possible prior to surgery. The best method of achieving this is use of general anesthesia. The vasodilatation with general anesthesia combined with use of hyperventilation to increase pO2 and decrease pCO2 is extremely effective in reducing intraocular pressure and no other systemic or topical therapy is required. If it is not possible to safely undertake a general anesthetic, intravenous acetazolamide may be considered an hour before surgery. Mannitol and oral glycerol are no longer recommended because of adverse systemic side effects. Remember acetazolamide is a diuretic, hence provision should be made for this side effect in theater. If all of the above are not possible, the final resort is to make an anterior chamber paracentesis and slowly release small amounts of aqueous from the paracentesis to bring the IOP gently down. This is absolutely a final resort and NOT the first option.

Surgical Step Traction suture.

Potential complication Full-thickness suture, tearing out, distorting closure.

How to avoid A traction suture is not a prerequisite for trabeculectomy surgery and it can be perfectly adequately completed in the vast majority of patients without such a suture. Most, however, prefer to use a suture in which case placement of the suture is the first consideration. A vast majority of surgeons place the suture in the cornea at 12'o-clock. Consideration may be given to the use of 3 and 9 o'clock or even 6'o-clock (see Fig. 4.1) traction suture(s).

Both of these options avoid a gaping effect on the scleral flap, which can cause aqueous flow from the anterior chamber and distort the anatomy.

If the cornea is perforated full thickness, during placement of the traction suture this should be easily identified by not only sensation but also the egress of aqueous. Simply withdraw the needle and hydrate the wound if need be and place the suture more superficially elsewhere. Should the anterior chamber have gone very shallow, simply wait and it will refill allowing the operation to proceed as usual.

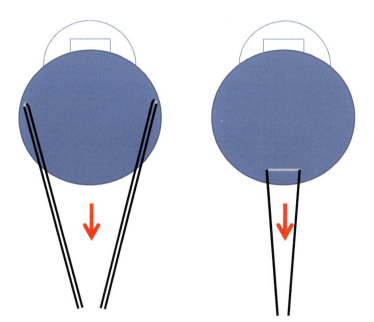

Fig. 4.1 (**a**) Traction sutures placed at 3 and 9 o'clock to avoid distortion of scleral flap. (**b**) Traction suture placed at 6 o'clock to avoid distortion of scleral flap

We recommend releasing the traction suture prior to entering the anterior chamber to avoid the risk of anterior chamber shallowing and difficulty closing the scleral flap due to countertraction (if the traction suture is in the 12 o-clock position).

Surgical Step Conjunctival incision and dissection.

Potential complication Incomplete dissection of Tenon's capsule from sclera.

This can lead to difficulty in dissecting the scleral flap, as the Tenon's tissue can make it difficult to judge the depth of the scleral flap. Releasable sutures can also become embedded in Tenon's which is adherent to the sclera, making them prone to snapping when trying to remove them.

How to Avoid Tenon's attaches approximately 0.5 mm behind the anatomical limbus. While dissecting, take the decision to take both the Tenon's and conjunctival tissue at the same time, or dissect each layer in turn. We find that a generous conjunctival opening at the limbus, enables easier and cleaner dissection of the Tenon's from the scleral bed. Should there be any adherent Tenon's capsule on the sclera, it is important to remove this by gentle scraping with a Tooke's knife, or similar instrument. Alternatively gentle cautery may shrink the adherent Tenon's for easy removal.

We find combined closure of the Tenon's and the conjunctiva at the limbus very helpful. If the Tenon's tissue is not brought forward at the limbus, then it can stick down posteriorly with scarring and cause the trabeculectomy to fail. Meticulous dissection at the start of the operation facilitates bilayered closure at the end.

Surgical step Conjunctival incision and dissection.

Potential complication Conjunctival buttonholes.

How to avoid Our standard technique is a fornix-based conjunctival flap. After the conjunctiva and Tenon's tissue has been dissected from the limbus, try to only grasp Tenon's tissue, either by rolling the limbal tissue backward over your forceps and so the Tenon's tissue is presented anteriorly, or by sliding a pair of toothed forceps underneath the Tenon's and grasping it from the under surface. This enables you to hold the "meaty" part of the Tenon's tissue and avoids accidental buttonhole of the conjunctiva when grasping both tissues together.

Some patients do however have very friable conjunctiva, and no matter how careful the dissection, conjunctival buttonholes may occur. Should a conjunctival button hole arise, it can be cut out if sufficiently anterior and enough tissue is available to be brought down to the limbus after the buttonhole has been excised. If the buttonhole is posterior, then we would ordinarily repair with a purse-string suture, of either 10/0 vicryl or nylon. Both these sutures have their merits. Vicryl is absorbable and due to the "vicrylitis" or tissue inflammation, encourages tissue healing. The healing, however, may be overaggressive and encourage scarring of the trabeculectomy. The nylon suture is only slowly absorbable, so may need removal at some stage. It is, however, less inflammatory for the tissues. Care must be taken to gently close the buttonhole, so as not to cheese-wire the tissue and create an extension of the original buttonhole. Completion of the suture from the undersurface of the conjunctiva ensures very good burying of the knot and fewer problems.

Surgical Step Cytotoxic application.

Potential Complication Thin-walled cystic bleb.

How to Avoid We advocate, as part of the Moorfields Safe Surgery technique, that a large area of cytotoxic is applied more posteriorly (Dhingra and Khaw 2009). To achieve this, Tenon's tissue is grasped at the limbal end of dissection, to keep it away from mitomycin C (MMC) and avoid contact of MMC with the conjunctiva. MMC soaked sponges are placed on the scleral bed, to give a large, posterior treatment area. Any excess MMC that has washed up at the limbus, is dabbed, during the 3-min treatment period. The sponges are then removed and the scleral bed is irrigated copiously with 20 ml of balanced salt solution (BSS). A large posterior treatment area is important, as it promotes diffuse posterior flow of aqueous and we believe may help prevent a "ring of steel" forming.

Surgical Step Cautery.

Potential Complication Focal thinning of sclera with aggressive cautery.

How to Avoid Although cautery is important to stop bleeding from episcleral and scleral vessels, aggressive cautery can cause focal scleral thinning, and irregular thickness to the scleral flap. Most bleeds do stop of their own accord, when given time. Another trick to reduce bleeding is to use topical 0.1 % epinephrine. The vasoconstriction decreases vascularity in the operative field and aids in the cessation of bleeding.

Surgical Step Scleral flap dissection.

Potential Complication Thin scleral flap: Full-thickness hole in scleral flap.

How to Avoid Thin scleral flaps are trouble. Sutures cheese-wire through them. They are difficult to close and can lead to anterior leaks and hypotony.

The key is recognition on the operating table. First, if there is an area of thin sclera, try and avoid this and move the site of the flap, laterally or medially to an area of healthier sclera.

If one does inadvertently create a full-thickness hole in the scleral flap, it can be subtle and we always recommend checking for leaks. Use of 2 % fluorescein after the flap has been sutured closed and the anterior chamber refilled to a physiological pressure with BSS via the paracentesis helps considerably in this respect. If a full-thickness hole is detected, then this should be closed with either a patch of Tenon's (autograft), or tutoplast at the time of surgery.

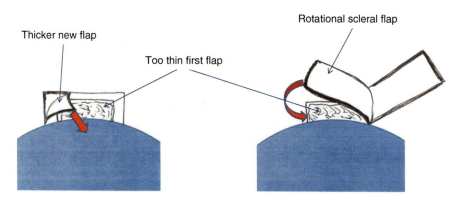

Fig. 4.2 (**a**) Dissection of a larger, thicker scleral flap, which incorporates the original thin scleral flap. (**b**) Dissection of a rotational scleral flap, which covers over the original thin scleral flap

If the flap is very thin overall, one can cut a flap around the original flap (see Fig. 4.2a), at a deeper depth, thus incorporating the original thin flap. This a good option, as normal anatomy is retained, it facilitates good flap closure and the position of the trabeculectomy remains optimal.

An alternative is to move to a new site.

Finally, if the leak is persistent and material scarce, a rotational scleral flap may be fashioned and folded over the original thin scleral flap (see Fig. 4.2b).

Surgical Step Scleral flap dissection.

Potential Complication Thick scleral flap: Valving.

How to Avoid Valving is the phenomenon that occurs when drainage only occurs on applying pressure behind the scleral flap. It is because there is no overlap of the side arms of the scleral flap and the sclerostomy (see Fig. 4.3a, b).

In order to detect valving, it is important to check drainage at the time of surgery. Once the sclerostomy and peripheral iridectomy are created, the scleral flap should be folded down, but not sutured down and the anterior chamber refilled with BSS via the paracentesis. If BSS is freely flowing out of the flap and the anterior chamber is spontaneously shallowing, then valving is not present and the flap can be closed. If on the other hand, no flow is seen from the back end of the flap once the anterior chamber is filled it indicates that aqueous will not drain from the flap, even if all the sutures have been removed. If this occurs two measures can be taken. The first is to cut-down the side arms more anteriorly. This however should not be undertaken, if the side arms are already very anterior, as it can lead to postoperative limbal leaks. The alternative is to enlarge the sclerostomy posteriorly. Once, one or both of these steps have been undertaken, then fold the flap back down and test again for flow. Once, you are confident that flow is present, then the flap can be sutured down.

Surgical Step Scleral flap dissection.

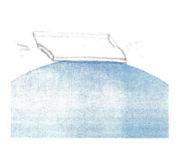
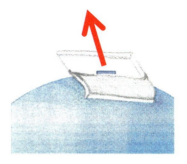

Fig. 4.3 (**a**) A valving effect is created due to lack of overlap between side arms of scleral flap and sclerostomy. (**b**) Overlap of side arms of scleral flap and sclerostomy, thus avoiding valving effect

Leak from full thickness incision   Leak sealed with box stitch

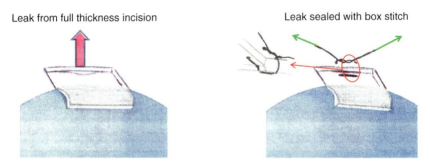

Fig. 4.4 (**a**) Creation of a full-thickness incision in sclera, when creating initial posterior scleral flap edge. (**b**) Repair of the full-thickness incision sutures, once scleral flap is completed

Potential Complication Thick scleral flap: Full-thickness initial incision. Persistent hypotony.

How to Avoid A full-thickness incision is not always spotted at the time of surgery and equally may not always lead to trouble. None-the-less it can result in persistent hypotony and the explanation only becomes clear on exploration of the operative site. A full-thickness incision most commonly occurs during the initial creation of the posterior flap edge, but full thickness can also be achieved with side arms and with enthusiastic flap dissection (both free hand and with the crescent knife). The principal method of avoidance is being aware that this can happen and lead to problems. If it does occur, suturing the defect is the simplest approach. In order to repair the defect, finish creating the scleral flap; this enables complete visualization of the full-thickness defect and avoids distortion while suturing it closed. It is important that the full-thickness incision is completely clear and then closed with either interrupted or box suture(s) (see Fig. 4.4a, b).

 If adequate dissection is not performed then the subsequent dissection may either cut the suture out or be completely distorted by the suture. The same principal applies if undertaking a revision. Take the whole operation down and explore using

2 % fluorescein. Suture the defect and then restore normal operative anatomy in your usual fashion.

Surgical Step Scleral flap dissection.

Potential Complication Premature anterior chamber entry.

How to Avoid This most usually happens at the anterior limit of sclera flap dissection. If it occurs, aqueous will be noticed at the scleral flap and the anterior chamber may shallow. A paracentesis is important for surgical control, so if there is not one already present and the anterior chamber has shallowed, insert a Rycroft cannula into the site of anterior chamber entry and fill the anterior chamber from here. Once the anterior chamber has deepened, create a paracentesis.

The site of premature entry can often be used to create the sclerostomy, it will otherwise require repair.

Surgical Step Scleral flap dissection.

Potential Complication Anterior drainage of aqueous, high anterior bleb with corneal epithelial disturbance.

How to Avoid The direction of aqueous flow is related to the scleral flap shape. Aqueous will preferentially follow the shortest route from sclerostomy to subconjunctival space. Figure 4.5 illustrates how this might vary with different flap shapes and why we prefer an oblong flap.

Surgical Step Sclerostomy.

Potential Complication Too small/too anterior: valving.

How to Avoid See section on valving above.

Surgical Step Sclerostomy.

Potential Complication Too large/too posterior.

How to Avoid When dissecting the scleral flap, correct identification of the blue-gray transition zone of the surgical limbus is key. This zone is approximately 1.2 mm and is due to the oblique interface of the sclera and cornea. Posterior to this zone is the opaque white sclera and anterior to it, is clear cornea.

When advancing from sclera to cornea, a sharply demarcated white line is encountered that roughly corresponds to the level of scleral spur. Next the tissue appears grayish over the trabeculum giving way to clear cornea at the level of Schwalbe's line. Therefore, to ensure entry into the anterior chamber, the incision must be in the anterior portion of this transition zone (Van Buskirk 1989).

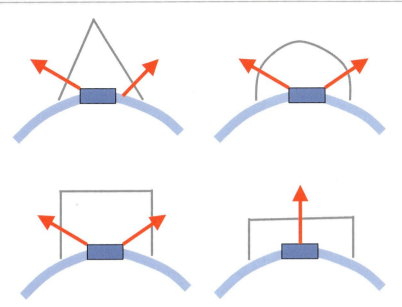

Fig. 4.5 Preferential flow of aqueous in direction of shortest path out of scleral flap. Different flap shapes influence direction of aqueous flow

Should the sclerostomy be made too posteriorly, the danger is catching the ciliary body tissue. This can lead to profuse bleeding, or even creation of a cleft. Should this situation arise the bleeding usually stops by closing the flap, allowing blood to drain externally, and simply waiting. In the unlikely event of a cleft being created this may need suturing to close.

Surgical Step Sclerostomy.

Potential Complication A partial thickness/shelved sclerostomy.

How to Avoid By definition, a sclerostomy is a full-thickness hole in the sclera. If using a scleral punch to create the sclerostomy, it is important to hold the punch vertically, to ensure a full-thickness bite of the sclera is taken. When the sclerostomy is full-thickness, a knuckle of iris tissue will often present itself, through the patent sclerostomy. If there is any doubt explore and enlarge.

Surgical Step Surgical peripheral iridectomy.

Potential Complication Bleeding.

How to Avoid The iris is supplied by anterior ciliary and long posterior ciliary arteries, which anastomose at the circulus arteriosus major and then supply the substance of the iris. The iris is a vascular structure and has the potential to bleed profusely on creation of a peripheral iridectomy. In the event of hemorrhage from the iris tissue, place the scleral flap down and refill the anterior chamber via the paracentesis and wait for the bleeding to stop. The elevated anterior chamber pressure acts as a tamponade to stop bleeding. If the bleeding is profuse, another alternative is to gently press on the back of the scleral flap and allow blood to drain out via the sclerostomy. This can, however, run the risk of prolonged hypotony. Washing blood out of the anterior chamber is not for the faint-hearted and we warn against cavalier removal of blood. If it is deemed necessary, tissue plasminogen activator (tPA) can be injected into the anterior chamber enabling blood clots to be removed more freely. There is a risk of rebleeding with anterior chamber washout. This risk is increased if tPA is used.

There is a shift in paradigm regarding the creation of a surgical peripheral iridectomy. Some surgeons advocate not performing surgical peripheral iridectomy in eyes that have deep anterior chambers and are not predisposed to the iris blocking the ostium (De Barros et al. 2009). However, the risk of iris obstruction will remain should the anterior chamber shallow in the absence of a peripheral iridectomy. While this can be controlled on the operating table, care must be taken when removing releasable sutures and massaging the bleb, in an outpatient setting.

Surgical Step Suturing of scleral flap.

Potential Complication Perioperative hypotony.

How to Avoid Sudden reduction in intraocular pressure and prolonged perioperative hypotony is best avoided since it may lead to suprachoroidal hemorrhage. A helpful step in prevention of prolonged hypotony is the use of preplaced scleral sutures (either releasable or fixed). These facilitate swift closure of the scleral flap and restore integrity of the eye. In eyes at higher risk of suprachoroidal hemorrhages or with advanced field loss it may be worth considering use of an anterior chamber maintainer to give greater stability of the anterior chamber.

Surgical Step Suturing of scleral flap.

Potential Complication Suture track leak.

How to Avoid This commonly happens with thin scleral flaps. It can also happen with full-thickness bites through the scleral flap, particularly when taking releasables through the base of the flap (limbal end). Recognition is important, and the use of 2 % fluorescein facilitates detection of leaks. In these circumstances first consider repositioning the sutures to stop the suture track leak. If this is not practical because the scleral flap is very thin and friable or repositioning of sutures is unlikely to help, it is important to remember that they often resolve and a temporary tamponade of the anterior chamber with viscoelastic or gas may be all that is indicated. Should the flap be torn by the suture then repair may be required as outlined in the section on scleral flap dissection.

Surgical Step Suturing of scleral flap.

Potential Complication Leakage from scleral flap edge.

How to Avoid Again detection is key and the use of 2 % fluorescein can be very helpful. Remedying a leak from the scleral flap edge may simply require additional fixed or releasable sutures. In cases, where the flap edge continues to leak, it is important to consider whether the anatomy of the flap has been distorted in some way. The simplest solution is to take down all scleral sutures, assess the scleral flap anatomy, and replace all the sutures again. Keep reviewing the situation in search of a solution, which is almost always possible. The final resort is to tamponade the anterior chamber with gas or viscoelastic to reduce flow out of the sclerostomy in the early postoperative period.

Surgical Step Suturing of scleral flap.

Potential Complication Postoperative hypotony.

How to Avoid This may be caused by loosening of one or more of the scleral sutures. We personally advocate placement of three releasable sutures to the scleral flap: one each to the nasal and temporal ends and one centrally (Dhingra and Khaw 2009). It is important to ensure that the sutures are tied tightly enough at the time of surgery and to detect any leaks at the time of surgery.

4.3 Early Postoperative Complications

Potential Complication IOP rise.

How to Manage This is the preferred early complication of trabeculectomy surgery simply because it ensures that you are in control of the eye and it is easily rectified. Too low a pressure is much more challenging. Removal of releasable sutures, laser suture lysis, bleb massage, and needling of the bleb are all tools to employ. As a very rough guide there is a window of about 6 weeks to establish a good surgical fistula in Caucasian eyes. This window is reduced in Asian eyes and still further reduced in African eyes.

It is also worth noting, that in the first 1–2 weeks, the trabeculectomy flap can be sealed shut with blood and massage often does not achieve flow of aqueous from the sclerostomy, or even precipitates bleeding into the anterior chamber. If the IOP is normal, then monitor and the clot will usually lyse within a couple of weeks, enabling establishment of aqueous flow.

We believe that the postoperative care is as important as the surgery during this window. Prior to enlisting patients for surgery, it is important to counsel them about frequent steroid use, frequent clinic visits, and bleb manipulations in clinic to ensure they understand what they are undertaking and that it requires full participation from their part. As is the case for successful repair in retinal detachment surgery, the first trabeculectomy has your best chance of achieving excellent IOP control for the patient long term. It is this window of opportunity that both you and your patient must commit to in order to ensure establishment of a functional surgical fistula. Review as often as required, manipulate the bleb as often as required, always being mindful of overdoing it and ending up with hypotony! Involvement of patients in this process is critical. In some carefully chosen instances they can even be enlisted in self-massage of the bleb. Subconjunctival injections of steroid and antimetabolite may be helpful, if the patient is showing signs of scarring and topical steroid use is essential.

The IOP can still be elevated, despite doing all you can to lower the IOP (e.g., bleb massage, removal/lysis of scleral flap sutures, subconjunctival injections of steroid, and antimetabolite). If this is the case, do not panic, as IOP does frequently goes through a "2 -month" spike (accordingly earlier in Asian and African eyes), from which complete recovery of bleb function and IOP are the norm, as the bleb remodels. This seems to be due to a natural healing process and does not necessarily need intervention (unless the IOP is unacceptably high).

Potential Complication Limbal leakage. Limbal or anterior drainage of aqueous can lead to hypotony, infection, and possibly early scarring and failure of the trabeculectomy.

How to Avoid and Manage Prevention is the key, water-tight closure at the limbus is important. As outlined above, we bring down Tenon's tissue to the limbus and secure it together with the conjunctiva to the anatomical limbus. Our standard method of closure is to use two purse-string sutures at the conjunctival edges and then horizontal mattresses sutures to close the center (see Fig. 4.6).

At the time of surgery, any leakage directly through the scleral flap or from the edges of the scleral flap should be identified and remedied on table. Small limbal leaks usually resolve spontaneously with no adverse effect (Henderson et al. 2004). If there is persistent hypotony, the patient should be taken back to theater and the trabeculectomy site explored for potential causes, such as very anteriorly placed side

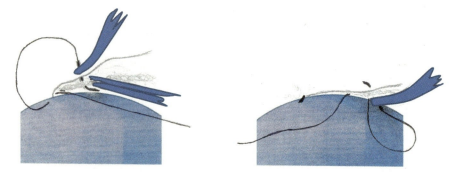

Fig. 4.6 Bilayered closure of Tenon and conjunctival tissue to the anatomical limbus

arms, or leakage through a thin scleral flap. It is also important to bear in mind that the patients may inadvertently be rubbing their eyes for iatrogenic reasons, such as loose sutures and eye drop allergies or intolerances. If this is the case, removing the cause if possible and advocating 24-h use of an eye shield may help stop the leak.

If there is dehiscence of the conjunctiva from the limbus, this should be taken back to theater and resutured straight away.

Potential Complication Hypotony (no conjunctival leakage).

How to Avoid and Manage It is important to ascertain the underlying cause of the hypotony and whether this is related to the surgery itself or to ocular risk factors for hypotony. Hypotony in relation to the surgery may be due to loose scleral flap sutures, full-thickness hole in the scleral flap, full-thickness scleral incision when creating the scleral flap, or even the patients rubbing their eyes due to ocular irritation. The commonest ocular-related risk factors for postoperative hypotony are high myopia and uveitis.

It is important to monitor these patients closely for resolution and to intervene in a timely manner if revision is needed. Our advice is to have a low threshold for revision in cases of hypotony, particularly in the presence of choroidals and hypotony maculopathy. If there is hypotony with the presence of a shallow anterior chamber, atropinizing the eye may allow the anterior chamber to deepen. Injecting a tamponade into the anterior chamber is a sound way of temporizing while awaiting resolution (for example, in the case of suture track leakage or high myopia). The tamponade may be an ophthalmic viscosurgical device (OVD) or gas (isovolumetric SF_6 or C_3F_8). The principal risk with such tamponades is a swing of the IOP a few hours after the injection to an extremely high IOP requiring release of the tamponade. Patients should be warned of this risk and given clear instructions regarding where to attend for immediate attention. The choice of tamponade is dependent on how profuse the leak is (the more profuse, the more viscous the OVD) and the surgeon's preference.

If there is hypotony in the context of a deep anterior chamber, with no choroidals or hypotony maculopathy, then it may be better to closely observe the patient for resolution of hypotony. Patients should be advised to rest and wear a shield over the eye especially during sleep. In particular rubbing of the eye, Valsalva maneuvers, and bending with the head dependent should be avoided, since there is a risk, not only of the leak being perpetuated but also of suprachoroidal hemorrhage.

In cases where hypotony is present, with a flat bleb, for example, in uveitics, it is important to keep the patient on high-dose topical steroid, as there may be poor flow of aqueous to maintain the surgical fistula due to temporary shutdown of the ciliary body.

Potential Complication Hyphema.

How to Avoid and Manage The blood may come from the iridectomy site or from the scleral flap site. It is important to note that these usually spontaneously clear remarkably quickly and resolve in most eyes. Thus rest is the first and foremost treatment. Consideration should be given to any contributory systemic factors, aspirin or anticoagulant use which may be amenable to intervention.

If the intraocular pressure is elevated in the context of hyphema, medical management may be the best option. The scleral flap may be sealed with clot and manipulation may restart active bleeding. Once the hyphema has resolved, it is, of course, extremely important to establish good flow through the trabeculectomy flap.

If medical therapy fails to control the intraocular pressure sufficiently, an anterior chamber washout may be required. It is worth considering an injection of tPA into the anterior chamber (see perioperative complications: hyphema). Oral tranexamic acid can also be used, to prevent rebleeding, when evacuating the clot.

Potential Complication Suture irritation.

How to Avoid and Manage Meticulous closure of the conjunctiva, ensuring all sutures are buried with trimmed ends, helps to avoid this problem. Nevertheless, despite the utmost care, suture irritation can still occur. All proud ends and redundant sutures can be trimmed or removed; for others reassurance and the promise of removing the conjunctival sutures 3–4 weeks from the date of surgery is usually sufficient. We endeavor to remove all conjunctival sutures 3–6 weeks after surgery in order to avoid subsequent irritation and the risk of bleb-related infection.

Potential Complication Snuff out.

How to Avoid and Manage Snuff out or wipe out of vision is a rare devastating complication (Costa et al. 1993). It is irreversible and typically occurs in patients with end-stage glaucoma. It is important to counsel patients thoroughly before embarking upon surgery and this is one of the rare complications to include in the discussion. As with all consultations it is important to present the relative risks of procedures and the rationale for intervention.

Although there is no evidence base as to why this occurs it has been hypothesized that sudden changes in intraocular pressure may contribute to this phenomenon. General anesthetic has been suggested as beneficial for those with end-stage glaucoma as there is no direct pressure on the optic nerve from the volume of the sub-Tenon's or peribulbar anesthesia and the intraocular pressure is lowered prior to ocular decompression. The use of an anterior chamber maintainer may also be considered to minimize sudden changes in intraocular pressure.

It should be noted that we have seen rare cases where the vision has been markedly decreased (even to NPL) postdecompression and yet has subsequently recovered over a few days. Thus visual loss on the first postoperative day, although serious, is not necessarily final.

Potential Complication Visual acuity decrease.

How to Avoid and Manage A majority of patients will experience loss of up to one line of acuity immediately posttrabeculectomy surgery. This can be due to a number of reasons including the new IOP, anterior chamber cells (red or white!), and corneal epitheliopathy. The most common reason, however, is irregular astigmatism from the flap. This has been well documented and takes up to 1 year to resolve completely (Hayashi et al. 2000). Simply waiting is almost always sufficient.

4.4 Late Postoperative Complications

Potential Complication Scarring, IOP rise.

How to Manage This is the most common complication of trabeculectomy surgery. If simply a clinical observation in the presence of adequate IOP and no glaucoma progression, then conservative management is indicated. If accompanied by a mild pressure rise and the patient previously responded, was compliant with, and tolerated previous topical ocular hypotensive therapy, then the resumption of drop treatment is usually adequate to retain glaucoma control. The next option frequently considered is needling revision of the bleb, usually with adjunctive cytotoxic and steroid therapy. In essence this is simply puncturing and slicing a hole(s) through the scar tissue to reestablish the surgical fistula. There is little evidence in the literature concerning needling, largely because of the very varied clinical population in whom it is performed with variation in age, time after surgery, diagnosis, type of bleb morphology, precipitation of failure (cataract surgery, uveitis, other ocular surgery, etc.), technique, and many other factors (Rotchford and King 2008). Success is variable and case selection is crucial. For the patient, the postoperative care can be as involved as the trabeculectomy and, with variable success rates, it is important to consider whether the patient definitely needs the needling revision or not. If you decide to proceed, ensure you perform gonioscopy to check that the internal ostium of the sclerostomy is not completely plugged with iris tissue. It is also important to consider the external ocular environment, the conjunctival morphology, and scleral flap prior to proceeding with needling revision.

Once you are happy that you have restored aqueous flow sufficiently, you may consider giving a subconjunctival injection of 5-fluorouracil (5-FU) and steroid.

The next possible approach to a scarred bleb is to consider trabeculectomy revision. This can either be the same site revision or a second trabeculectomy at a different site.

A final option is to consider other surgeries such as a drainage tube or cyclodiode ciliary body ablation.

Potential Complication Bleb dysesthesia.

How to Manage Bleb dysesthesia occurs due to disruption of the natural lid contour over the globe. Patients may complain of varying degrees of discomfort. Symptoms of bleb dysesthesia can vary from an awareness of the bleb, to constant discomfort, symptoms of exposure keratopathy, and even bubble formation and audible clicking, particularly in those with 360° exuberant blebs.

Counseling in these patients is important, as many patients are able to tolerate the symptoms, particularly in mild cases if they understand the cause. It is always worth trying a course of preservative-free ocular lubricants in the first instance, but these are not always effective.

A variety of approaches can be tried:

1. Injection of autologous blood (Smith et al. 1994)
2. The use of Palmberg sutures to limit the bleb (Palmberg and Zacchei 1996)
3. Revision of the bleb, with a patch graft (Clune et al. 1993)
4. Limiting incisions (Rossiter et al. 1999)

In the instance of persistent dysesthesia in the presence of a diffuse functional trabeculectomy our own approach is to undertake limiting incisions laterally and medially to the scleral flap. The cut edges can be "tacked" down to the scleral bed with sutures to limit the bleb.

For those patients with "high" domed blebs that cause intractable ocular discomfort, revision and bleb excision can give temporary relief, but the blebs commonly recur over time. Our own approach is to excise, completely seal with a patch graft, and insert an aqueous shunt to control the intraocular pressure.

Do note that none of these measures are suitable for an overdraining bleb causing hypotony. Please see the section on hypotony.

Potential Complication Cystic leaking bleb, endophthalmitis.

How to Manage It is important to remember that many blebs leak intermittently without the cognizance of the ophthalmologist. The majority do not come to harm. When considering whether to revise or observe, full consideration should be given to the patient's ocular, personal, and social environment. For example, one may be more likely to revise if the patient suffers from chronic infections, lives in an unsuitable home environment, self-neglects, or has restricted access to health care. If these concerns are present, it is better to revise than observe.

It is important to have a full discussion with the patient of the risks and ensure the understanding of seriousness of condition. If one gauges that the patient has a poor understanding of the situation, then a revision should be done.

It is a good idea to reinforce patient education, either in the form of patient information leaflets on bleb-related infection or with the help of a nurse counselor.

We also endeavor to give patients a supply of prophylactic topical antibiotics, which they are asked to commence immediately if they develop symptoms of bleb-related infection and are unable to reach expert review within an hour. The patient is asked to start these immediately and seek ophthalmic care as soon as possible, if they develop signs of an infection.

Potential Complication Hypotony in the presence of a deep anterior chamber.

How to Manage Hypotony is not just a figure, but a figure combined with signs. Signs of pathological hypotony include permanently or intermittently blurred vision. For example, vision may be blurred in the morning or when standing for prolonged periods. Permanent blurring or fluctuating vision, folds at the macula, or choroidals are signs that the eye needs attention. It is important to seek out an underlying cause that may require urgent attention, such as leaking bleb, retinal detachment, or uveitis.

If the eye is symptomatic, you have to either consider reducing outflow, by either using a tamponade in the anterior chamber or surgical revision. Use of a tamponade is really to buy time, before taking them to the operating theater.

If the patient is phakic, cataract surgery may produce enough inflammation to result in sufficient scarring to reverse the hypotony. In borderline cases, this can be a good measure, otherwise revision is the best and most definitive option. It should be noted that reversal of hypotony is often not immediate after cataract surgery.

Potential Complication Bleb-related infection.

How to Manage This can occur at any time point after surgery. In a meta-analysis we have done of ten publications in which the occurrence of infection in 4346 trabeculectomies has been reported over time, the incidence of bleb-related infection is approximately 0.5 % per year (Katz et al. 1985; Wolner et al. 1991; Greenfield et al. 1996; Higginbotham et al. 1996; Mochizuki et al. 1997; Uchida et al. 2001; DeBry et al. 2002; Muckley and Lehrer 2004; Shigeeda et al. 2006; Sharan et al. 2009). It is important to counsel all patients using verbal and written information with special attention to those with cystic or leaking blebs. Patients should be advised to obtain emergency eye care as soon as possible if a bleb-related infection is suspected, as time to treatment is critical (see Fig. 4.7).

All departments have a protocol to treat bleb-related infection and so we are not going to talk about antibiotic regimes. The point we would like to highlight is that

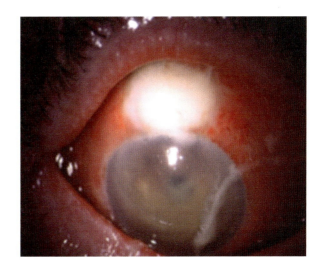

Fig. 4.7 Photograph of bleb-related infection, displaying classic "white on red" sign (Photograph taken by Ms. Poornima Rai, Consultant Ophthalmologist, Moorfields Eye Hospital, London)

steroids are critical to the visual outcome (Kangas et al. 1997). The inflammatory reaction precipitated by the infection can have devastating effects on the retina. We inject intravitreal dexamethasone at the same time as intravitreal antibiotics and commence patients on topical steroids and antibiotics immediately and oral steroids 12–24 h after intravitreal injections. The exception to the rule is suspicion of a fungal infection, in which case steroids should be withheld.

Potential Complication Progression of cataract.

How to Manage The incidence of cataract formation is 10–61 % after trabeculectomy surgery (Mathew and Murdoch 2011). It is not known why there is such a dramatic increase in cataract formation. The etiology is thought to be multifactorial. It is an age-old debate as to whether cataract surgery should be performed before or after trabeculectomy surgery and which way round is better for trabeculectomy survival. If trabeculectomy surgery is performed before, it is important to counsel patients regarding the risk of cataract progression. Please see section on coexistence of cataract.

Potential Complication Glaucoma progression despite controlled intraocular pressure.

How to Manage One can expect a continued rate of attrition of the ganglion cells even after surgery. In addition to normal attrition with age there may be ongoing loss during the immediate postoperative period. This may cause progressive visual field changes, which eventually plateau out. There is, however, a small subgroup of patients who continue to progress despite what appears to be optimum pressure control. This is a heart-sink moment for most clinicians. Two immediate questions to consider are

1. Is the IOP sufficiently low compared to the preoperative pressure at which they were advancing?
2. Is there sufficient control of IOP throughout the day?

If the answer to both the above questions is "Yes", then vascular and other factors need to be considered. If the patient is taking systemic antihypertensive therapy it is important to consider 24-h blood pressure monitoring (Graham and Drance 1999). If there are nocturnal dips in blood pressure a change in therapy may eliminate these and halt glaucoma progression. *Gingko biloba* may improve blood flow to the optic nerve head; it does not affect the IOP (Rhee et al. 2001). There is very little evidence regarding its efficacy.

Conclusion

This chapter is a practical guide for anticipation, prevention, and management of common and sight threatening complications of trabeculectomy surgery. Reported results of this well-established operation are happily improving over time and success proportions in excess of 90 % at 1 year and 80 % at 2 years are not uncommon (Kirwan et al. 2013). While there is still plenty of room for improvement, the operation is becoming much more predictable. Our aim has been to provide a framework for considering complications of trabeculectomy surgery. We hope it is helpful for anticipation, prevention, and management of complications in your own practice.

References

Broadway DC, Grierson I, Stürmer J, Hitchings RA. Reversal of topical antiglaucoma medication effects on the conjunctiva. Arch Ophthalmol. 1996;114(3):262–7.

Casson RJ, Riddell CE, Rahman R, et al. Long-term effect of cataract surgery on intraocular pressure after trabeculectomy. Extracapsular extraction versus phacoemulsification. J Cataract Refract Surg. 2002;28:2159e64.

Chen PP, Weaver YK, Budenz DL, et al. Trabeculectomy function after cataract extraction. Ophthalmology. 1998;105:1928e35.

Clune MJ, Shin DH, Oliver MMG, et al. Partial thickness scleral patch graft revision of trabeculectomy. Am J Ophthalmol. 1993;115:818–20.

Costa VP, Smith M, Spaeth GL, et al. Loss of visual acuity after trabeculectomy. Ophthalmology. 1993;100:599–612.

Crichton AC, Kirker AW. Intraocular pressure and medication control after clear corneal phacoemulsification and AcrySof posterior chamber intraocular lens implantation in patients with filtering blebs. J Glaucoma. 2001;10:38e46.

De Barros DS, Da Silva RS, Siam GA, et al. Should iridectomy be routinely performed as a part of trabeculectomy? Two surgeons' clinical experience. Eye. 2009;23:362–7.

DeBry PW, Perkins TW, Heatley G, et al. Incidence of late-onset bleb-related complications following trabeculectomy with mitomycin. Arch Ophthalmol. 2002;120:297–300.

Dhingra S, Khaw PT. The moorfields safer surgery system. Middle East Afr J Ophthalmol. 2009;16:112–5.

Ehnrooth P, Lehto I, Puska P, et al. Phacoemulsification in trabeculised eyes. Acta Ophthalmol Scand. 2005;83:561e6.

Graham SL, Drance SM. Nocturnal hypotension: role in glaucoma progression. Surv Ophthalmol. 1999;43(Suppl 1):S10–6.

Greenfield DS, Suner IJ, Miller MP, et al. Endophthalmitis after filtering surgery with mitomycin. Arch Ophthalmol. 1996;114:943–9.

Hayashi K, Hayashi H, Oshika T, Hayashi F. Fourier analysis of irregular astigmatism after trabeculectomy. Ophthalmic Surg Lasers. 2000;3:94–9.

Henderson HW, Ezra E, Murdoch IE. Early postoperative trabeculectomy leakage: incidence, time course, severity, and impact on surgical outcome. Br J Ophthalmol. 2004;88:626–9.

Higginbotham HJ, Stevens RK, Musch DC, et al. Bleb-related endophthalmitis after trabeculectomy with mitomycin C. Ophthalmology. 1996;103:650–6.

Kangas TA, Greenfield DS, Flynn Jr HW, et al. Delayed –onset endophthalmitis associate with conjunctival filtering blebs. Ophthalmology. 1997;104:746–52.

Katz LJ, Cantor LB, Spaeth GL. Complications of surgery in glaucoma. Early and late bacterial endophthalmitis following glaucoma filtering surgery. Ophthalmology. 1985;92:959–63.

Kiire CA, Mukherjee R, Ruparelia N, et al. Managing antiplatelet and anticoagulant drugs in patients undergoing elective ophthalmic surgery. Br J Ophthalmol. 2014;98:1320–4.

Kirwan JF, Lockwood AJ, Shah P, et al. Trabeculectomy in the 21st century: a multicentre analysis. Ophthalmology. 2013;120:2532–9.

Kotecha A, Spratt A, Ogunbowale L, et al. Intravitreal bevacizumab in refractory neovascular glaucoma. Arch Ophthalmol. 2011;129:145–50.

Mathew RG, Murdoch IE. The silent enemy: a review of cataract in relation to glaucoma and trabeculectomy surgery. Br J Ophthalmol. 2011;95:1350–4.

Mochizuki K, Jikihara S, Ando Y, et al. Incidence of delayed onset infection after trabeculec-tomy with adjunctive mitomycin C or 5-fluorouracil treatment. Br J Ophthalmol. 1997;81: 877–83.

Muckley ED, Lehrer RA. Late-onset blebitis/endophthalmitis: incidence and outcomes with mito-mycin C. Optom Vis Sci. 2004;81:499–504.

Palmberg P, Zacchei AC. Compression sutures: a new treatment for leaking or painful filtration blebs. Invest Ophthalmol Vis Sci. 1996;37:s444.

Park HJ, Kwon YH, Weitzman M, et al. Temporal corneal phacoemulsification in patients with filtered glaucoma. Arch Ophthalmol. 1997;115:1375e80.

Rebolleda G, Munoz-Negrete FJ. Phacoemulsification in eyes with functioning filtering blebs: a prospective study. Ophthalmology. 2002;109:2248e55.

Rhee DJ, Katz LJ, Spaeth GL, et al. Complementary and alternative medicine for glaucoma. Surv Ophthalmol. 2001;46:43–55.

Rossiter JD, Godfrey SJ, Claridge KG. A case of a 360 degree exuberant trabeculectomy bleb. Eye. 1999;13:369–79.

Rotchford AP, King AJ. Needling revision of trabeculectomies bleb morphology and long-term survival. Ophthalmology. 2008;115:1148–53.

Sharan S, Trope GE, Chipman M, et al. Late-onset bleb infections: prevalence and risk factors. Can J Ophthalmol. 2009;44:279–83.

Shigeeda T, Tomidokoro A, Chen YN, et al. Long-term follow-up of initial trabeculectomy with mitomycin C for primary open-angle glaucoma in Japanese patients. J Glaucoma. 2006;15:195–9.

Siriwardena D, Kotecha A, Minassian D, et al. Anterior chamber flare after trabeculectomy and after phacoemeulsification. Br J Ophthalmol. 2000;84:1056–7.

Smith MF, Magauran R, Doyle JW. Treatment of postfiltration bleb leak by bleb injection of autol-ogous blood. Ophthalmic Surg. 1994;25:636–7.

Swamynathan K, Capistrano AP, Cantor LB, et al. Effect of temporal corneal phacoemulsi-fication on intraocular pressure in eyes with prior trabeculectomy with an antimetabolite. Ophthalmology. 2004;111:674e8.

Uchida S, Suzuki Y, Araie M, et al. Long-term follow-up of initial 5-fluorouracil trabeculectomy in primary open-angle glaucoma in Japanese patients. J Glaucoma. 2001;10:458–65.

Van Buskirk EM. The anatomy of the limbus. Eye. 1989;3:101–8.

Wolner B, Liebmann JM, Sassani JW, et al. Late bleb-related endophthalmitis after trabeculectomy with adjunctive 5-fluorouracil. Ophthalmology. 1991;98:1053–60.

Wong TT, Khaw PT, Aung T, et al. The Singapore 5-fluorouracil trabeculectomy study: effect on intraocular pressure control and disease progression at 3 years. Ophthalmology. 2009;116:175e84.

K. Sheng Lim, David Steven, and Francis Carbonaro

5.1 Background

Tube and plate glaucoma drainage devices have been in general use since AC Molteno introduced his first glaucoma drainage device (GDD) in 1969 (Molteno 1969). For much of their history, these devices have been implanted in eyes that had failed trabeculectomy. However, more recent studies, notably the Tube versus Trabeculectomy Study's (TVT 5-year result) (Gedde et al. 2012) have suggested that tube surgery may be appropriate at much earlier stages of glaucoma. Certainly, in the instance of aphakia, secondary glaucoma resulting from surgery, or any other cases where there is excessive conjunctival scarring, primary tube surgery may well be the best long-term option.

The use of tube surgery declined during the 1980s, when surgeons encountered many visually devastating complications, which brought about the regulation of tube surgery in many large ophthalmic centers. However, as the complication mechanisms became better understood, and means to avoid them were developed, tube surgery's popularity made a resurgence in the late 1990s, and in some centers it has become more widely performed than trabeculectomy (Lim et al. 1998).

In this chapter we will review the current rate of complications associated with glaucoma tube surgery, describe the mechanisms that cause these complications, and detail precautions against, and management of, complications should they occur. Table 5.1 lists the contemporary glaucoma drainage devices that are most commonly used.

K. Sheng Lim • D. Steven
St Thomas Hospital, London, UK

F. Carbonaro (✉)
Mater Dei Hospital, Msida, Malta
e-mail: franciscarbonaro@gmail.com

Table 5.1 Contemporary glaucoma drainage devices

	Year of introduction	Tube diameter/ material	Plate size/material	Resistance mechanism
Molteno	1969	0.63 mm OD 0.30 mm ID Silicone	135 mm² Polypropylene	None
Baerveldt	1990	0.63 mm OD 0.30 mm ID Silicone	200, 250, 350, 425, 500 mm² Silicone	None
Ahmed	1993	0.63 mm OD 0.30 mm ID Silicone	185 mm² FP7 model silicon plate with silicone valve in polypropylene box	Venturi valve

OD outside diameter, *ID* inside diameter

5.2 Evaluating Glaucoma Drainage Device Results

Most GDDs have been developed in a virtual publication vacuum, with little available data to substantiate manufacturers' claims for flow performance or biocompatibility (Prata et al. 1995). Clinical data are largely restricted to uncontrolled retrospective case series (Krawczyk 1995) with variable follow-up and differing definitions of surgical success. Evaluation is further complicated by the heterogeneity of inclusion criteria. Series include a variable proportion of complex cases, such as neovascular glaucoma, in which there is a higher risk of filtration failure.

Overall success rates, in terms of IOP control, appear similar between devices (Table 5.2), with a reasonably high proportion of cases achieving a final IOP in the target range at 1 year after surgery. Half to two-thirds of these cases still require glaucoma medications, however, target IOPs in the low teens (≤ 16 mmHg) may be more realistic in terms of preventing disease progression than commonly adopted target levels (≤ 21 or 22 mmHg).

Another important caveat concerns attrition rates, or continued increments in the proportion of filtration failures with lengthening postoperative follow-up. Again, evaluation is difficult, with few series including either long-term data or survival analysis (Mills et al. 1996) (Table 5.2). Mills et al. reported a 10 % failure rate per postoperative year in a series including longer-term follow-up for single and double plate Molteno tubes. Extrapolating from this would suggest that many GDDs have a functional lifespan of less than 5 years before failure though fibrous encapsulation. However, the 5-year data from the Tube vs. Trabeculectomy (TVT) study found a 10 % failure rate per year for the first 3 years, and an average of 5 % per year for the subsequent 2 years, which may indicate better long-term results with less complex cases (Gedde et al. 2012).

5.2.1 Tube Use, Tube Type, and Complication Risk

Clinical series reporting GDD procedures are characterized by frequent problems in addition to filtration failure (Table 5.3), with overall complication rates

Table 5.2 Success rates of current GDDs

Type	Investigator	Year	Diagnosis	No. of eyes	Follw-up (months) mean ± SD	Success criteria	Success rate w/o medication	Success rate with medications
Molteno								
SP and DP	Mills et al. (1996)	1996	Mixed (25 % neovascular)	77	44[a]	IOP ≤22 mmHg and NFC[b]	23 %	34 %
SP	Mermoud et al. (1993)	1993	Neovascular	60	24.7±13.4	IOP ≤21 mmHg and NFC[b]	17 %	20 %
SP	Heuer et al. (1991)	1992	Mixed (no neovascular)	50	14.9±8.9	5 ≤IOP ≤21 mmHg and NFC[b]	10 %	40 %
DP				52	16.4 ± 6.8		12 %	63 %
SP	Minckler et al. (1988)	1988	Mixed (50 % neovascular)	90	17.6	IOP ≤21 mmHg and NFC[b]	7 %	40 %
Ahmed valve	Coleman et al. (1995)	1995	Mixed	60	9.3[a]	IOP <22 mmHg[c,d] and NFC[b]	NA	NA (78 %)[e]
	Coleman et al. (1997)	1997	Penetrating keratoplasty[f]	31	16[a]	IOP <22 mmHg[c,d] and NFC[b,g]	26 %	39 %
	Coleman et al. (1997)	1997	Pediatric-mixed	24	16.3±11.2	IOP <22 mmHg[c,d] and NFC[b]	33 %	38 %
	Barton et al. (2014) (ABC group)	*2014*	*Mixed*	*106*	*36*	*IOP <22 mmHg[c] and NFC[b,g]*	*20 %*	*84%[h]*
	Christakis et al. (2013) (AvB study)	*2013*	*Mixed*	*124*	*36*	*IOP <18 mmHg IOP >5 mmHg[c] and NFC[b,g]*	*13 %*	*57 %[h]*
Krupin disk	The Krupin Study Group (1994)	1994	Mixed	50	25.4±2.4	IOP ≤19 and NFC[b]	47 %	33 %
	Fellenbaum et al. (1994)	1994	Mixed	25	13.2	6 ≤ IOP ≤21 and NFC[b]	28 %	36 %

(continued)

Table 5.2 (continued)

Type	Investigator	Year	Diagnosis	No. of eyes	Follow-up (months) mean ± SD	Success criteria	Success rate w/o medication	Success rate with medications
Baerveldt 200, 250, 350, 500 mm²	Seigner et al. (1995)	1995	Mixed	103	13.6±0.9	5 ≤ IOP ≤22 and NFC[b]	45 %	27 %
200, 350, 500 mm²	Sidoti et al. (1995)	1995	Neovascular	36	15.7±7.2	6 ≤ IOP ≤21 and NFC[b]	33 %	17 %
350 mm² 500 mm²	Lloyd et al. (1994)	1994	Mixed	37 36	15.5±4.8 14.1±5.4	6 ≤ IOP ≤21 and NFC[b]	14 % 36 %	70 % 47 %
Diameters mixed/not specified.	*Barton et al. (2014) (ABC group 3 years)*	*2014*	*Mixed*	*100*	*36[a]*	*IOP <22 mmHg[c] and NFC[b,g]*	*33 %*	*72%[h]*
350 mm²	*Christakis et al. (2013) (AvB study)*	*2013*	*Mixed*	*114*	*36*	*IOP <18 mmHg IOP >5mmHg[c] and NFC[b,g]*	*33 %*	*86%[h]*
350 mm²	*Gedde et al. (2009) (TvT 3 year study)*	*2009*	*Mixed*	*107*	*36*	*IOP <21 mmHg IOP >5 mmHg[c] and NFC[b,g]*	*56 %*	*85 %*

[a]Median follow-ups in months
[b]With no further glaucoma surgery or devastating complication
[c]Or reduction of >20 % if preoperative IOP >22 mmHg
[d]Data from same patients may appear in more than one of these three series
[e]Total success rate only
[f]Concurrent or prior
[g]Including graft failure
[h]Defined as 100 % − %(reported failure rate). The figure therefore includes qualified successes

NFC no further complications, *Molteno SP* Molteno single plate, *Molteno DP* Molteno double plates, *ABC study* Ahmed Baerveldt Comparison study (Barton et al. 2014), *AvB study* Ahmed versus Baerveldt study (Christakis et al. 2013), *TvT study* tube versus trabeculectomy study (Gedde et al. 2009)

Table 5.3 Cumulative complication rates among currently used GDDs

Implants	Ahmed valve (1990s)	Ahmed valve (recent)	Baerveldt implant (1990s)	Baerveldt implant (recent)
Studies	Coleman 1995	ABC 2014[a]	Lloyd 1994	ABC 2014[a]
	Coleman 1997	AvB 2013[b]	Sidoti 1995	AvB 2013[b]
	Coleman 1997		Smith 1993	TvT 2009[c]
			Siegner 1995	
n =	115	267	249	354
Complication category	Rate (%)	Rate (%)	Rate (%)	Rate (%)
Choroidal effusion	14.00 %	6.00 %	23.00 %	9.90 %
Tube erosion, occlusion, malposition	17.30 %	7.90 %	15.60 %	9.30 %
Shallow anterior chamber	3.50 %	7.10 %	16.50 %	9.60 %
Persistent corneal edema/decompensation	3.50 %	8.60 %	11.60 %	11.60 %
Persistent diplopia/motility disorder	3.50 %	8.60 %	21.00 %	6.20 %
Iritis/uveitis	1.70 %	4.90 %	3.60 %	5.10 %
Hyphema	0.00 %	2.20 %	11.00 %	2.80 %
Vitreous hemorrhage	3.50 %	1.10 %	7.00 %	1.10 %
Encapsulated/encysted bleb	3.50 %	5.60 %	1.60 %	1.40 %
Retinal/choroidal detachment	0.00 %	1.50 %	5.00 %	2.50 %
Phthisis bulbi	0.00 %	0.00 %	2.40 %	1.40 %
Aqueous misdirection/malignant glaucoma	0.90 %	0.70 %	2.00 %	1.40 %
Suprachoroidal hemorrhage	3.50 %	0.00 %	0.80 %	1.40 %
Other complications[d]	4.30 %	6.40 %	6.00 %	9.30 %
n = Postoperative complications per patient tested[e]	**0.6**	**0.6**	**1.3**	**0.7**
% of tested patients experiencing complications.	**60–70 %[f]**	**45 %[a,b]**	**60–70 %[f]**	**51%[a,b,c]**

[a]*Ahmed Baerveldt comparison study* (Barton et al. 2014)
[b]*Ahmed* versus *Baerveldt study* (Christakis et al. 2013)
[c]*Tube* versus *Trabeculectomy study* (Gedde et al. 2009)
[d]Complications whose rate was <2 % in all categories
[e]Note that some patients had more than one complication
[f]Estimate: (Heuer et al. 1991; Siegner et al. 1995)

typically around 60–70 % (Heuer et al. 1991; Siegner et al. 1995). While partly attributable to the complex nature of cases typically selected for implantation, the range of complications observed also reflects design and material inadequacies inherent in contemporary GDDs. The origin of most complications can be traced to just two fundamental mechanisms: poor flow control and suboptimal material biocompatibility.

In the past, tube surgery was performed on patients with advanced forms of glaucoma, such as neovascular glaucoma, which carried a higher risk of complications. In recent times, surgeons have increasingly used tubes to treat less advanced patients, resulting in a lower rate of complications recorded in recent studies.

5.3   Major Postoperative Complications and Their Mechanisms

The risk profile of major postoperative complications following the implantation of a glaucoma drainage device (GDD) is similar to those that follow a trabeculectomy. Drainage issues give rise to "early hypotony" and the subsequent "hypertensive" phases, whereas a range of mechanical and inflammatory problems can beset the tube's interactions with the anterior chamber. Further complication categories, including eye motility and infections, are associated either with the tube or the plate.

5.3.1   Poor Flow Control

Insufficient internal flow regulation and uncontrolled extrinsic leakage have all been implicated in the problems associated both with excessive aqueous outflow in the early postoperative stages and with the impediments to drainage that can follow. The different complication risk profiles of Ahmed and Baerveldt implants reflect important differences in their design and the way they manage hypotony.

5.3.1.1   GDD and Flow Control Mechanisms

Since Molteno's original device, minimizing rates of hypotony has been the main drive behind modifications to GDDs and implantation techniques. This is typically experienced over the first two postoperative months, until formation of a fibrous capsule around the plate offers sufficient resistance to aqueous outflow. Hypotony is associated with a catalog of early and late complications (Table 5.3). Anterior chamber flattening is especially hazardous in the context of GDD implantation because contact with the tube element can cause significant damage to the lens and cornea. In addition, all GDD devices are susceptible to a later elevation of IOP brought about by bleb encapsulation. GDDs can be categorized into those with no internal resistance mechanism, such as the Baerveldt implant, and those which aim to provide set internal flow resistance, such as the Ahmed valve.

Early independent examinations of the flow characteristics for Ahmed, Baerveldt, and other GDDs revealed a significant discrepancy between observed function, and the manufacturers' claims for flow resistance (Prata et al. 1995). The Krupin valve appeared not to close after initial opening in perfusion tests conducted at physiological flow rates. Resistance values also varied considerably between devices from the same manufacturer, indicating deficiencies in quality control (Porter et al. 1997). However, subsequent flow examinations (Eisenberg et al. 1999; Francis 1998) showed that the Ahmed valve might indeed have a more consistent opening and closing pressure. Clinically, hypotony was still reported in 5–20 % of cases after Ahmed GDD implantation (Coleman et al. 1997; Coleman 1997). Inconsistencies in flow control continue to be observed in some Ahmed valves, prompting some surgeons to perform flow-testing with saline pre-implantation to ensure the valve opening and closing pressures remain with appropriate boundaries (Jones et al. 2013).

5.3.1.2 Early Hypotony and Its Consequences

The primary outcome of hypotony is a shallow or flat anterior chamber. The shallowing of the anterior chamber greatly increases the risk of even a correctly positioned tube touching the corneal endothelium or the iris, which ultimately increases the risk of corneal decompensation, or uveitis, respectively. Hypotony also increases the chances of tube occlusion (Bailey and Sarkisian 2014). Severe flattening of the anterior chamber can bring the iris and cornea into contact. Although it has been shown not to cause devastating complications itself (Fiore 1989), iridocorneal touch can result in adhesion, cataracts, and endothelial cell loss, which put the cornea at greater risk of decompensation (Hosoda et al. 2013).

Choroidal effusions, which involve the filling of the suprachoroidal space with serum, are commonly associated with postoperative hypotony and flat anterior chambers. For the most part, they are asymptomatic and resolve once IOP is normalized. However, if choroidal effusions should expand and touch one another, "kissing choroidals" may cause irreversible damage. Inflammation of capillaries with serous choroidal effusions may trigger suprachoroidal hemorrhage. The use of GDDs, as opposed to trabeculectomy, generally appears to reduce the risk of choroidal effusion (Gedde et al. 2009; Schrieber and Liu 2015). Chronic hypotony can also lead to macular edema with resulting decrease in vision and if this occurs management to reverse the hypotony should be instilled.

5.3.1.3 Bleb Encapsulation

Long-term management of postoperative IOP relies on the formation of a bleb, or fibrous capsule around the end plate. A successful bleb must not adhere to the plate, but form a space around it which filters out aqueous humor. Early postoperative hypotony is expected to correct itself following the proliferation of fibroblasts around the plate (Schwartz et al. 2006).

However, it is not uncommon for the filtering bleb to overcompensate, leading to elevated IOP, which typically presents any time between 2 and 12 postoperative months. The greater the surface area and the thinner the wall of fibroblasts, the lesser the resistance to aqueous outflow. The bleb's inflammatory response to the arrival of aqueous into the end plate may initiate a positive feedback system, since thickened capsule walls inevitably increase intraocular (and bleb) pressure, intensifying the stress response of the fibroblasts, causing them to thicken. Although the risk of postoperative hypotony is less with Ahmed implants, they are markedly more susceptible (Chen and Palmberg 1997) to bleb encapsulation, possibly due of their smaller size and rougher surface material (Choritz et al. 2010).

5.3.2   Complications of the Tube and Anterior Chamber

The tube's implantation technique is the foremost factor in the successful drainage of the anterior chamber. Whether or not it is the result of poor flow control, hypotony increases the risk of tube-related complications being initiated in the shallowed anterior chamber, since tube tips are far more likely to come into contact with the iris or cornea.

5.3.2.1   Leakage Around the Tube

All the commonly used devices feature a round silicone anterior chamber tube with a diameter of between 0.56 and 0.63 mm (Table 5.2). The recommended technique for insertion is through a paracentesis track created by either a 22 or 23 gauge (0.65 mm) hypodermic needle. Debate over the optimum needle gauge continues (Coleman et al. 1995), but insertion often requires considerable manipulation. Even then, the tube to paracentesis fit can be poor, and uncontrolled leakage external to the tube is common. More rarely, the implant tube has been shown to erode at its entry point to the anterior chamber, resulting in fluid leakage (Al-Torbak 2001) (Fig. 5.1).

5.3.2.2   Hyphema

Hyphema generally occurs when vessels are damaged as the tube enters the anterior chamber, whether because of a posterior insertion hitting the iris root or abnormal vessels angle vessels, such as in neovascular glaucoma. Bleeding will be exacerbated in hypotony. It is important, especially in cases of neovascular glaucoma, to examine the angle prior to surgery to look for angle new vessels or peripheral

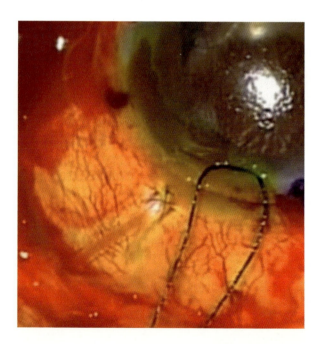

Fig. 5.1 Fluorescein dilution by aqueous leakage around the tube after implantation

Practical Tip: Tube Entry with a 25G Needle

- Start 2 mm from the limbus with a smooth single entry initially in the plane of the sclera then angle forward parallel with the iris plane once half of the bevel is in the sclera.
- Ensure a single movement without retraction or advancement (as this can create a false pocket).
- Enlarge the track slightly on exit to aid with initiating the tube entry.
- Check for watertight fit with 2 % fluorescein, suture adjacent to the tube if leaking.
- Persistent leaks may be stopped by plugging with sub-Tenon's tissue.
- Anterior vitrectomy should be performed if there is any chance of vitreous in the AC, usually from previous complicated cataract surgery.

Fig. 5.2 Perioperative hyphema in a neovascular glaucoma after tube insertion into the anterior chamber. The bleeding is from the angle blood vessels

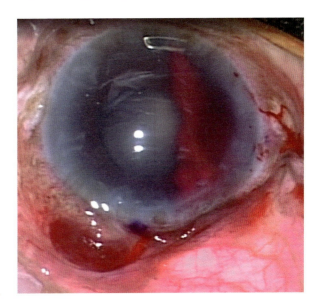

anterior synechiae in the area of planned insertion and either avoid the affected areas or avoid vessels by inserting more anteriorly (Fig. 5.2).

5.3.2.3 Tube Blockage by Iris, Vitreous, or Cornea

During the implantation of a GDD, it is very important that the bevel of the tube is cut upwards toward the corneal endothelium. This will eliminate, or at least reduce, the risk of iris tissue occluding the tube at its entry site. Should iris occlusion occur at a later date, it may be necessary to perform a secondary iridectomy or to re-site the tube. Argon laser can sometimes be used to retract iris tissue from around the tube as well.

The blockage of the tube by vitreous in the anterior chamber or sulcus space is a commonly encountered problem. Generally, if the eye has (a) had prior partial vitrectomy, (b) had any loss of vitreous during cataract surgery, or (c) had even a suggestion of vitreous strands coming into the anterior chamber during tube surgery, then it is necessary to perform an anterior vitrectomy at the time of tube surgery. This will reduce the risk of vitreous incarceration into the tube.

The chances of corneal endothelial touch can be greatly mitigated by good surgical technique. It is advisable to implant a tube entry site well into the pigmented trabecular meshwork area; and it is important that entry plane of the needle is at least parallel to the iris plane. Should corneal endothelial touch occur postoperatively, it is essential that the tube is revised, either by re-siting or trimming. Prolonged corneal touch will cause the failure of its endothelial cells in the long run.

5.3.2.4   Corneal Decompensation

Persistent corneal edema has been cited as the most frequent postoperative complication for GDDs that appears after 12 months (Topouzis et al. 1999). Corneal preservation relies on the health of its endothelial cells, which lie between it and the anterior chamber. High IOP causes the loss and morphological change of these cells, whereas excessive shallowing of the anterior chamber following GDD implantation brings the corneal endothelium into contact with the tube, causing long-term mechanical trauma (Alvarenga et al. 2004). The risk of this complication is greatly elevated among patients with preexisting corneal pathologies or grafts (Gedde et al. 2009).

To minimize the risk of any anterior chamber part of the tube touching corneal endothelium, it is essential to make sure that the tube lies much closer to the iris than the cornea (Fig. 5.3).

5.3.3   Subconjunctival and Explant Complications

5.3.3.1   Diplopia

Diplopia is a fairly common problem, although in the TVT trial, a similar rate of diplopia is encountered in both trabeculectomy and tube surgery. The first generation

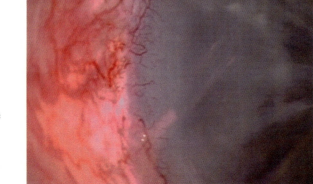

Fig. 5.3 Tube in the anterior chamber too close to endothelium and subsequent intermittent rubbing caused localized corneal edema around the tube entry site

of Baerveldt tube implants, whose plates did not feature a perforating anchoring hole, encountered a very high proportion of patients with postoperative diplopia. Since the introduction of perforating holes in the later Baerveldt plates, the diplopia risk has been greatly reduced, but remains significantly higher than that of the Ahmed implant. This reflects the greater size of the Baerveldt end plate. It is important to thoroughly assess the patient preoperatively, and warn the patient of this potential complication. The diplopia is often self-limiting and may be observed in the early postoperative phase (Rauscher et al. 2009). Persistent cases may often be managed with prismatic correction but occasionally squint surgery or even explantation of the device may be required.

5.3.3.2 Tube or Plate Erosion

In general, the tube in the subconjunctival space needs to be covered either by a long needle track, by a scleral flap created as per trabeculectomy, or else a patch graft formed either from donor pericardium, sclera, or cornea to reduce the risk of erosion. Once the tube is properly covered, the risk of erosion is less than 2 % in the reported literature. It is most common adjacent to the limbus as this is where the greatest angulation of the tube occurs and where overriding eyelid movement is greatest (Fig. 5.4) (Panarelli et al. 2016). Micromotion of the tube may also play a role. This can be reduced by the placement of one to two mattress sutures of either 10-0 nylon or 9-0 prolene to anchor tube to the sclera.

5.3.3.3 Poor Biocompatibility

In the context of GDD implantation, biocompatibility describes how safely the synthetic material interfaces with living tissues. Suboptimal biocompatibility is manifest in an array of complications including early fibrinous occlusion of the tube, corneal endothelial failure, tube migration, extrusion, and fibrous encapsulation leading to filtration failure. Protein adhesion and micromotion are key elements in the mechanism of these complications.

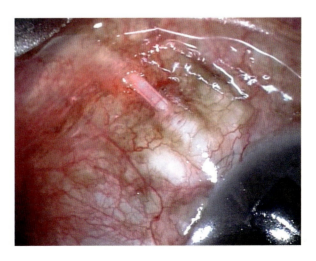

Fig. 5.4 Eroded tube despite previous pericardium patch graft

Elastomeric silicone (polydimethylsiloxane) remains the most commonly used material in current GDDs. Silicone, PMMA, and other hydrophobic polymers used in GDDs have a relatively high binding affinity for plasma and interstitial fluid proteins such as albumin, IgG, and fibrinogen all of which are adsorbed within hours of implantation (Pitt et al. 1988). Cellular adhesion, cytokine release, and chronic inflammation are thought to be mediated via elements of this protein film (Tang and Eaton 1995).

Continuing low grade inflammation is exacerbated by micromotion, or microscopic shearing of the implant, relative to the surrounding tissues. Plate elements of contemporary GDDs often restrict the movements of the extraocular muscles, either directly or through adhesions with septal elements of the orbital tissues. Even where this does not produce a frank motility disturbance, it is likely that shear forces transmitted through the relatively rigid materials used in GDD construction produce significant micromotion. In rabbit experiments, fenestration of the Baerveldt GDD significantly reduced fibrous encapsulation thicknesses compared with unfenestrated controls, as was observed at explantation 6 months postoperatively (Jacob-LaBarre et al. 1995). In addition to causing subconjunctival fibrosis after GDD implantation, micromotion effects may be transmitted through the tube directly to the anterior chamber, where it may cause corneal endothelial cell loss. The co-occurrence of these effects with perioperative endothelial damage is possibly a major contributor to corneal endothelial failure.

Progressive fibrous encapsulation limits the filtration life of all contemporary GDDs. Whether due to poor flow control, or suboptimal biocompatibility, the mechanism that causes the inexorable progression from low grade inflammation, to subconjunctival fibrosis has not yet been adequately addressed.

5.4   Managing Postoperative Complications

5.4.1   Managing Hypotony

The flow chart (Fig. 5.5) illustrates the management of patients with hypotony post-tube surgery. The key component of assessing whether intervention is required is to determine whether the anterior chamber is formed, or if there is any other associated retinal complication. Should there be a flat anterior chamber, the tube needs to be tied; otherwise there will be long-term consequences, including corneal endothelial failure as well as suprachoroidal hemorrhage. If the anterior chamber is only slightly shallow, then an intervention is only justified in cases of maculopathy or suprachoroidal effusion. It will then be necessary to administer injections of a cohesive viscoelastic such as Healon. If there is no indication of these conditions, despite a shallow anterior chamber, then the patient can be reviewed very closely on a weekly basis until their condition improves. It may also be good clinical practice to add atropine 1 % twice a day to the eye, in order to reduce the risk of aqueous misdirection.

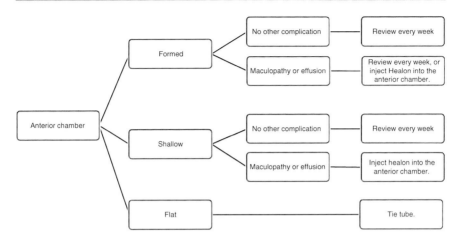

Fig. 5.5 A flowchart for the management of early hypotony

	Iris	*Vitreous*	*Cornea*
Precautionary measure	Cut the tube bevel upwards towards the cornea.	Note whether partial vitrectomy has occurred, or whether vitreous strands are observed in the anterior chamber.	Implant the tube deep in the trabecular meshwork, and, entry plane of the needle must be parallel to the iris plane.
If Blocked	Secondary iridectomy, or re-siting of the tube.	If any of the above occur, an anterior vitrectomy is necessary.	Re-site or trim the tube. If retracted tube extender can be utilised.

Fig. 5.6 Management of tube-related complications

5.4.2 Managing Tube Blockage/Retraction and Hyphema

Figure 5.6 summarizes the main causes of tube blockage, preventative measures, and recourse if the tube is blocked. Most hyphemas can be observed but if extensive, then blocking the tube intracameral tissue plasminogen activator (3–5 μg diluted to a total of 0.1 ml with sterile water) (Panarelli et al. 2016) together with topical mydriatics and steroids may dissolve the clot. Persistence of blockage requires anterior chamber washout in theater.

5.4.2.1 Tube Retraction
If the tube is suspected to have retracted significantly into the sclerostomy tract causing complete occlusion of the tube, this must be associated with the absence of drainage into the bleb over the plate. Should this be confirmed, a tube extender (New World Medical, California, USA) is a useful tool to overcome this complication (Fig. 5.7).

5.4.2.2 Viscoelastic Injection Technique
When postoperative hypotony results in a shallow anterior chamber, it is necessary to inject Healon into the anterior chamber. In the office, this can be achieved with the use of topical anesthetic and a needle piercing the cornea; 150–200 μl is typically administered, depending on the desired volume of the anterior chamber.

Fig. 5.7 Tube extender (New World Medical, California, USA) used to extend a previously retracted tube

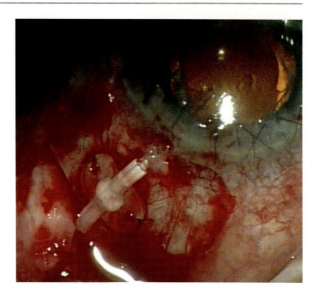

Practical Tip: Viscoelastic Injection
- Insulin syringe (1 ml with needle), preloaded with 150 μl of Healon and bend needle for easier access
- Topical anesthesia with tetracaine
- Betadine 5 % installation into the conjunctival sac
- Assistant to hold the eyelid may be required
- A slit lamp Healon injected via the peripheral cornea into the anterior chamber
- Recheck the IOP in 30 min and review in 5–7 days

5.4.2.3 Tube Tie Technique

Where the hypotony is severe or persistent despite multiple viscoelastic injections into the anterior chamber, it is best to halt the flow of aqueous from the anterior chamber by tying off the tube. Once the free end of the tube is accessed through an incision in the cornea, it is tied off, typically with an 8-0 prolene suture. Multiple permanent ties of prolene are advised in the AC portion of the tube, ideally with an intraluminal 3-0 prolene suture. These permanent sutures can be loosened at a later stage using an argon laser.

Practical Tip: Tube Tie Technique:
- Perform in theater with general anesthesia if possible.
- If the tube is long enough to externalize, then proceed as follows (if the tube within the AC is too short to be exernalized, then a conjunctival peritomy will be required, the tube is removed from the AC, tied off, and then replaced).
- Place AC maintainer and perform paracentesis with an MVR blade.
- Incise cornea over tube as in figure.

Figure: incision to externalize tube.

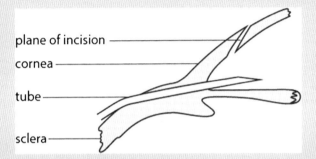

- Externalize the tube by hooking out with a Sinskey hook.
- 3.0 supramid or prolene can be placed within the tube lumen if not already in position.
- Two to three 8.0 prolene sutures can then be tied over the tube and the tube replaced in the AC and the conjunctival incision sutured, 3.1.1 tie.
- The 8.0 prolene sutures can be lasered under direct visualization with a gonioscopy lens when increased flow is desired (argon laser settings 0.5 s, 200 μm, 150–200 mW), typically after at least 6 weeks.

5.4.3 Managing Choroidal Effusions and Hemorrhage

If the IOP is within acceptable limits, choroidal effusions can be observed as they usually resolve without treatment beyond steroid drops and cycloplegics (Schrieber and Liu 2015). If the intraocular pressure is low, then this should be addressed as shown in Fig. 5.4. If the choroidal detachments are touching, "kissing choroidals" or the anterior chamber flat, then surgical intervention is required.

Suprachoroidal hemorrhage can be an intraoperative complication, termed expulsive hemorrhage, or more commonly can occur postoperatively, when it is known as delayed suprachoroidal hemorrhage (DSCH). More frequently after tube

Practical Hint: Draining Choroidal Effusions

- Place AC maintainer (in some situations this alone may be enough to allow some resolution of effusions).
- Place sclerotomies in area of choroidals 4–8 mm back from limbus.
- Open the conjunctiva and then make radial incisions gradually through sclera with number 15 blade.
- As the suprachoroidal space is entered the serosanguinous effusion should start draining.
- Gently massage the globe with a cotton bud as this may assist in drainage, which should be continued until fluid egress ceases.
- The sclerotomies can be left open to drain more fluid, the conjunctiva securely closed with 7.0 vicryl suture.

surgery than trabeculectomy in most series DSCH presents with a sudden onset of pain, loss of vision, shallowing of the anterior chamber, and increased IOP. Other symptoms can also include nausea (Vaziri et al. 2015). They can often be left to clear, especially if peripheral, but there is no clear guidance from the literature with some reporting resolution of large hemorrhages with conservative management (Chu and Green 1999), and good results described with early intervention (Pakravan et al. 2014). If the hemorrhage is massive with retinal apposition, a flat anterior chamber or severe persistent pain, then drainage and reformation of the anterior chamber can be attempted. This can be done early, within the first 24–36 h, or delayed by 1 week to allow clot dissolution to occur. Vitrectomy may be required if an associated retinal detachment develops. Visual outcomes are generally poor, so recognition and, where possible, mitigation of risk factors is important (Jeganathan et al. 2008).

Table: Risk Factors for DSCH

- High preoperative pressure
- Severe early postoperative hypotony
- Previous intraocular surgery
- Long axial length
- Aphakia
- Anticoagulation
- Systemic hypertension

5.4.3.1 Malignant Glaucoma

Malignant glaucoma, or aqueous misdirection syndrome, is rare, but can present at any time postoperatively, typically with a shallow anterior chamber and high intraocular pressure. Most cases respond to medical treatment with IOP lowering agents and topical mydriatics and steroids. Disruption of the anterior hyaloid face with

Nd:YAG laser can be tried in pseudophakic patients, peripheral to the IOL. If these measures are unsuccessful, then surgical intervention is required in the form of core vitrectomy, often combined with cataract extraction in phakic patients (Kaplowitz et al. 2015).

5.4.3.2 Managing Tube Exposure

Exposure of the tube places the patient at risk of endophthalmitis and therefore all cases should be revised. The tube must be covered with a patch graft of donor pericardium, sclera, or cornea and this then covered with conjunctiva. The risk of further conjunctival breakdown is minimized by the use of a rotational flap of conjunctiva, usually from the conjunctival fornix and this is therefore recommended (Grover et al. 2013). The other option is to use a tube extender to divert to adjacent subconjunctival space with relatively healthier conjunctiva (Fig. 5.7 and 5.8).

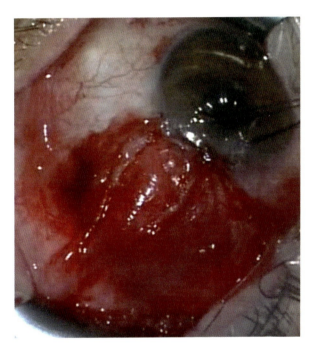

Fig. 5.8 Rotational conjunctival graft covering the tube extender and pericardial patch

Practical Tip: Covering an Exposed Tube
- Perform surgery under GA if possible as can be uncomfortable under LA.
- Instill preoperative apraclonidine 1 % and adrenaline into the conjunctival sac.
- Place a 7.0 silk traction suture in the cornea.
- Excise a small rim of conjunctiva and scrape exposed sclera to improve adhesion of graft.
- Place a 10.0 nylon mattress suture over the tube to reduce micromovement of the tube.

- Cover the tube with a patch graft (such as tutoplast pericardium), anchoring with a 10.0 nylon suture anteriorly and a mattress suture across the graft.
- Dry conjunctiva and mark out a pedical flap of sufficient size to rotate to and cover conjunctival defect.
- Incise flap and rotate into position, suturing securely with 10.0 nylon.
- Administer subconjunctival cefuroxime and dexamethasone and give dexamethasone and antibiotic drops postoperatively.

5.4.3.3 Managing Plate Erosion

Erosion of the plate through the conjunctiva is rare and when it occurs it usually requires explantation. Preventive measures include care to ensure that the wings of the Baerveldt plate are behind the rectus muscles, otherwise the plate can come to lie superficially under the conjunctiva where it is more prone to erode. Firm sutures are needed to secure the plate to the sclera and to avoid eye rubbing postoperatively.

5.4.4 Managing Bleb Encapsulation

There is little evidence to suggest that MMC use intraoperatively in the region of the plate or 5-FU injections postoperatively are beneficial in the long term (Law 2008). One study to report positive effects with these two combined used an older version of the Ahmed valve and a surgical technique that may also have contributed to lower intraocular pressure (Alvarado et al. 2008). Revision of thick-walled blebs with excision of fibrous tissue has been described in a small case series (Eibschitz-Tsimhoni et al. 2005). Molteno advocates an "anti-inflammatory fibrosis suppression" regimen consisting of oral prednisone, colchicine, and NSAIDs in three divided doses per day in the early postoperative period, started in the first 3 weeks and continued for 4–8 weeks (Vote et al. 2004; Fuller et al. 2002). This has not been widely used or studied due to concerns about the possible systemic side effects. Ultimately, a significant proportion of tube patients require topical IOP lowering agents. Unlike after trabeculectomy surgery this is not usually a sign of impending or total bleb failure.

Conclusion

Postoperative complications are frequently associated with tube surgeries, the most common ones are hypotony, tube touching endothelium, tube occlusion, tube erosion, and bleb encapsulation. Most of these complications can be minimized with careful surgical techniques or perioperative testing of the flow characteristics through the tubes, but once encountered, most need urgent rectifications, or long-term sequelae will prevail.

References

Al-Torbak A. Transcorneal tube erosion of an Ahmed valve implant in a child. Arch Ophthalmol. 2001;119(10):1558.

Alvarado JA, et al. Ahmed valve implantation with adjunctive mitomycin C and 5-fluorouracil: long-term outcomes. Am J Ophthalmol. 2008. 146(2):276–84.

Alvarenga LS, et al. The long-term results of keratoplasty in eyes with a glaucoma drainage device. Am J Ophthalmol. 2004;138(2):200–5.

Bailey AK, Sarkisian SR. Complications of tube implants and their management. Curr Opin Ophthalmol. 2014;25(2):148–53.

Barton K, et al. Three-year treatment outcomes in the Ahmed Baerveldt comparison study. Ophthalmology. 2014;121(8):1547–57.e1.

Chen PP, Palmberg PF. Needling revision of glaucoma drainage device filtering blebs. Ophthalmology. 1997;104(6):1004–10.

Choritz L, et al. Surface topographies of glaucoma drainage devices and their influence on human tenon fibroblast adhesion. Invest Opthalmol Vis Sci. 2010;51(8):4047.

Christakis PG, et al. The Ahmed versus Baerveldt study. Ophthalmology. 2013;120(11):2232–40.

Chu TG, Green RL. Suprachoroidal hemorrhage. Surv Ophthalmol. 1999;43(6):471–86.

Coleman AL. Initial clinical experience with the Ahmed glaucoma valve implant in pediatric patients. Arch Ophthalmol. 1997a;115(2):186.

Coleman AL, et al. Initial clinical experience with the Ahmed glaucoma valve implant. Am J Ophthalmol. 1995;120(1):23–31.

Coleman AL, et al. Clinical experience with the Ahmed glaucoma valve implant in eyes with prior or concurrent penetrating keratoplasties. Am J Ophthalmol. 1997b;123(1):54–61.

Eibschitz-Tsimhoni M, et al. Incidence and management of encapsulated cysts following Ahmed glaucoma valve insertion. J Glaucoma. 2005;14(4):276–9.

Eisenberg DL, et al. In vitro flow properties of glaucoma implant devices. Ophthalmic Surg Lasers Imaging Retina. 1999;30(8):662–7.

Fellenbaum PS, et al. Krupin disk implantation for complicated glaucomas. Ophthalmology. 1994;101(7):1178–82.

Fiore PM. The effect of anterior chamber depth on endothelial cell count after filtration surgery. Arch Ophthalmol. 1989;107(11):1609.

Francis B. Characteristics of glaucoma drainage implants during dynamic and steady-state flow conditions. Ophthalmology. 1998;105(9):1708–14.

Fuller JR, et al. Anti-inflammatory fibrosis suppression in threatened trabeculectomy bleb failure produces good long term control of intraocular pressure without risk of sight threatening complications. Br J Ophthalmol. 2002;86(12):1352–4.

Gedde SJ, et al. Three-year follow-up of the tube versus trabeculectomy study. Am J Ophthalmol. 2009;148(5):670–84.

Gedde SJ, et al. Treatment outcomes in the Tube Versus Trabeculectomy (TVT) study after five years of follow-up. Am J Ophthalmol. 2012;153(5):789–803 e2.

Grover DS, et al. Forniceal conjunctival pedicle flap for the treatment of complex glaucoma drainage device tube erosion. JAMA Ophthalmol. 2013;131(5):662–6.

Heuer DK, et al. Glaucoma update IV. In: Preliminary report of a randomized clinical trial of single plate versus double plate molteno implantation for glaucomas in Aphakia and Pseudophakia. Springer Science + Business Media; 1991. p. 244–9.

Hosoda S, et al. Ophthalmic viscoelastic device injection for the treatment of flat anterior chamber after trabeculectomy: a case series study. Clin Ophthalmol. 2013;7:1781–5.

Jacob-LaBarre JT, et al. Total integration of an ocular implant/prosthesis. Ophthalmic Plast Reconstr Surg. 1995;11(3):200–8.

Jeganathan VS et al. Risk factors for delayed suprachoroidal haemorrhage following glaucoma surgery. Br J Ophthalmol. 2008;92(10):1393.

Jones E, et al. Preimplantation flow testing of Ahmed glaucoma valve and the early postoperative clinical outcome. J Curr Glaucoma Pract. 2013;7(1):1–5.

Kaplowitz K, et al. Current concepts in the treatment of vitreous block, also known as aqueous misdirection. Surv Ophthalmol. 2015;60(3):229–41.

Krawczyk CH. Glaucoma drainage devices and the FDA. Ophthalmology. 1995;102(11):1581–2.

Law SK. A modified technique of Ahmed glaucoma valve implantation with adjunctive use of antifibrotic agents. Am J Ophthalmol. 2008;146(2):156–8.

Lim KS, et al. Glaucoma drainage devices; past, present, and future. Br J Ophthalmol. 1998;82(9):1083–9.

Lloyd MA, et al. Intermediate-term results of a randomized clinical trial of the 350- versus- the 500-mm2 Baerveldt implant. Ophthalmology. 1994;101(8):1456–64.

Mermoud A, et al. Motteno tube implantation for neovascular glaucoma. Ophthalmology. 1993;100(6):897–902.

Mills RP, et al. Long-term survival of molteno glaucoma drainage devices. Ophthalmology. 1996;103(2):299–305.

Minckler DS, et al. Clinical experience with the single-plate Molteno implant in complicated glaucomas. Ophthalmology. 1988;95(9):1181–8.

Molteno AC. New implant for drainage in glaucoma. Clinical trial. Br J Ophthalmol. 1969;53(9):606–15.

Krupin eye valve with disk for filtration surgery. Ophthalmology. 1994;101(4):651–8.

Pakravan M, et al. An alternative approach for management of delayed suprachoroidal hemorrhage after glaucoma procedures. J Glaucoma. 2014;23(1):37–40.

Panarelli JF, Nayak NV, Sidoti PA. Postoperative management of trabeculectomy and glaucoma drainage implant surgery. Curr Opin Ophthalmol. 2016;27(2):170–6.

Pitt WG, Grasel TG, Cooper SL. Albumin adsorption on alksyi chain derivatized polyurettianes. Biomaterials. 1988;9(1):36–46.

Porter JM, Krawczyk CH, Carey RF. In vitro flow testing of glaucoma drainage devices. Ophthalmology. 1997;104(10):1701–7.

Prata JA, et al. In vitro and in vivo flow characteristics of glaucoma drainage implants. Ophthalmology. 1995;102(6):894–904.

Rauscher FM, et al. Motility disturbances in the tube versus trabeculectomy study during the first year of follow-up. Am J Ophthalmol. 2009;147(3):458–66.

Schrieber C, Liu Y. Choroidal effusions after glaucoma surgery. Curr Opin Ophthalmol. 2015;26(2):134–42.

Schwartz KS, Lee RK, Gedde SJ. Glaucoma drainage implants: a critical comparison of types. Curr Opin Ophthalmol. 2006;17(2):181–9.

Sidoti PA, et al. Experience with the Baerveldt glaucoma implant in treating neovascular glaucoma. Ophthalmology. 1995;102(7): p. 1107–18.

Siegner SW, et al. Clinical experience with the Baerveldt glaucoma drainage implant. Ophthalmology. 1995;102(9):1298–307.

Tang L, Eaton JW. Inflammatory responses to biomaterials. Am J Clin Pathol. 1995;103(4):466–71.

Topouzis F, et al. Follow-up of the original cohort with the Ahmed glaucoma valve implant11. The views expressed herein are those of the authors and are not the official opinions of the Department of the Navy, the Department of Defense, or the United States Government. Am J Ophthalmol. 1999;128(2):198–204.

Vaziri K, et al. Incidence of postoperative suprachoroidal hemorrhage after glaucoma filtration surgeries in the United States. Clin Ophthalmol. 2015;9:579–84.

Vote B, et al. Systemic anti-inflammatory fibrosis suppression in threatened trabeculectomy failure. Clin Exp Ophthalmol. 2004;32(1):81–6.

Printed by Printforce, the Netherlands

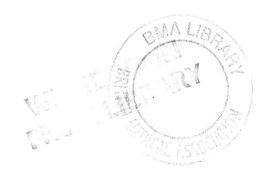